100 Questions & About Spine D

Rahul Jandial, MD

University of California, San Diego Medical Center—
Division of Neurosurgery
Burnham Institute for Medical Research—
Center for Neurosciences
Regenerative Medicine Program
La Jolla, CA

Henry E. Aryan, MD

University of California, San Francisco (UCSF)
Department of Neurological Surgery
Complex Spinal Reconstruction & Neurospinal Oncology
Neurosurgical Associates Medical Group
Fresno, CA

JONES AND BARTLETT PUBLISHERS
Sudbury, Massachusetts
BOSTON   TORONTO   LONDON   SINGAPORE

World Headquarters

Jones and Bartlett
Publishers
40 Tall Pine Drive
Sudbury, MA 01776
978-443-5000
info@jbpub.com
www.jbpub.com

Jones and Bartlett
Publishers Canada
6339 Ormindale Way
Mississauga, Ontario L5V 1J2
CANADA

Jones and Bartlett
Publishers International
Barb House, Barb Mews
London W6 7PA
UK

Jones and Bartlett's books and products are available through most bookstores and online booksellers. To contact Jones and Bartlett Publishers directly, call 800-832-0034, fax 978-443-8000, or visit our website www.jbpub.com.

Substantial discounts on bulk quantities of Jones and Bartlett's publications are available to corporations, professional associations,and other qualified organizations. For details and specific discount information, contact the special sales department at Jones and Bartlett via the above contact information or send an email to specialsales@jbpub.com.

The authors, editor, and publisher have made every effort to provide accurate information. However, they are not responsible for errors, omissions, or for any outcomes related to the use of the contents of this book and take no responsibility for the use of the products and procedures described. Treatments and side effects described in this book may not be applicable to all people; likewise, some people may require a dose or experience a side effect that is not described herein. Drugs and medical devices are discussed that may have limited availability controlled by the Food and Drug Administration (FDA) for use only in a research study or clinical trial. Research, clinical practice, and government regulations often change the accepted standard in this field. When consideration is being given to use of any drug in the clinical setting, the health care provider or reader is responsible for determining FDA status of the drug, reading the package insert, and reviewing prescribing information for the most up-to-date recommendations on dose, precautions, and contraindications, and determining the appropriate usage for the product. This is especially important in the case of drugs that are new or seldom used.

Production Credits
Executive Publisher: Christopher Davis
Production Director: Amy Rose
Associate Production Editor: Rachel Rossi
Associate Editor: Kathy Richardson
Associate Marketing Manager: Rebecca Wasley

Manufacturing Buyer: Therese Connell
Composition: Cape Cod Compositors, Inc.
Cover Design: Jon Ayotte
Printing and Binding: Malloy, Inc.
Cover Printing: Malloy, Inc.

Library of Congress Cataloging-in-Publication Data:
Jandial, Rahul.
    100 questions and answers about spine disorders / Rahul Jandial, Henry E. Aryan.
       p.   cm.
    Includes bibliographical references and index.
    ISBN-13: 978-0-7637-4988-0 (pbk.)
    ISBN-10: 0-7637-4988-5 (pbk.)
    1. Spine—Diseases—Popular works.   2. Spine—Diseases—Miscellanea.   I. Aryan, Henry E.
II. Title.   III. Title: One hundred questions and answers about spine disorders.
    RD768.J36   2008
    616.7'3—dc22
                                                                                2007031768
6048

Printed in the United States of America
11 10 09 08   10 9 8 7 6 5 4 3 2 1

To my mother, Sushma Jandial, for always encouraging me toward ambitions that benefit not only myself but, more importantly, others.

To my father, Satya Pal Jandial, for providing me with the fundamental pillars of pride and integrity on which one should build one's life.

—Rahul Jandial

To my parents, Hani and Aida, who taught me about duty and charity, without which life is hollow.

To my wife, Hala, whose support and steadfastness helped serve as a compass to navigate me throughout my career.

—Henry Aryan

Contents

Contents

Part 12: Spine Rehabilitation — 151

Questions 93–100 provide practical advice regarding therapy and lifestyle changes, such as:

- What are my limitations?
- How long do I have to wear my collar or brace?
- What about pain management?

As medicine and surgery have enjoyed a continued expansion of the number and variety of treatments that they can offer people with illness, a new challenge has arisen for both doctors and patients. This challenge has been to provide information that is actually meaningful. Such information would consist of more than just facts and statistics; it would constitute the distillation of the vast fund of current medical knowledge into specific information and advice that people can understand and incorporate into their own decisions. We have written this book with the intention of providing just such a resource in the hope that it might be of great value to both patients and the doctors who provide their care.

100 Questions & Answers About Spine Disorders provides introductory yet thorough medical information from which patients can gain insight into their illness and an understanding of the variety of treatment options that exist. We hope that, by acting as a supplemental educational reference for patients, it will allow clinicians to have a more open and comprehensive dialogue with those patients regarding their care. Our ultimate hope is that, for those who have diseases of the spine, this text will serve as a bridge to a more meaningful interaction with their care-givers and as a resource from which they can feel empowered for personal healing.

PART ONE

The Healthy Spine and Spinal Cord

What are the anatomy and function of the spine?

What are discs made of?

What happens to the spine as we age?

More . . .

1. What are the anatomy and function of the spine?

The spine is a unique part of the body that has complex architecture for a variety of functions. The spine must serve as rigid structural support that houses the **spinal cord** and has holes (foramen) from which nerves can exit and extend to different parts of the body and extremities. At the same time, it must be a movable and flexible construct that allows for neck and back movement. This dual purpose is satisfied by the spine being in bony segments (vertebrae) and having compressible segments (intervertebral discs) in between, allowing for both motion and stability. The amount of support versus mobility varies among the different regions of the spine. The spine in the neck (**cervical** spine) has a great amount of mobility, with little load-bearing function. However, the spine in the back (**lumbar** spine) can bear significant weight, but has less mobility. Furthermore, the spine is divided into alternating fixed and mobile segments. The fixed skull transitions into the flexible cervical spine. This, in turn, transitions to the fixed **thoracic** spine. The thoracic spine transitions to the flexible lumbar spine, which ultimately transitions to the fixed sacral spine in the hips.

The spine is not designed to be completely straight. In fact it has very important curves that help with load bearing and allow us to look straight and stand up straight. Kyphoses are curves that are concave anteriorly (if you are looking at a person from the side, the bulge of the curve would be pointing toward the back), and lordoses are curves that are concave posteriorly (if you are looking at a person from the side, the bulge of

The Healthy Spine and Spinal Cord

Spinal cord
the nervous system tissue that relays information to and from the limbs and the brain. It is located within the center of and protected by the vertebrae.

Cervical
the neck region. Specifically, there are seven cervical vertebrae in the human spine. They are numbered C1, C2, etc. The nerves that exit the spine in this region are responsible for movement and sensation in the arms and hands.

Lumbar
the low back region. Specifically, there are five lumbar vertebrae in the human spine. They are numbered L1, L2, etc. The nerves that exit the spine in this region are responsible for movement and sensation in the legs and feet.

Thoracic
the mid-back region. Specifically, there are twelve thoracic vertebrae in the human spine, each associated with a pair of ribs. They are numbered T1, T2, etc.

the curve would be pointing to the front). The cervical spine has a natural lordosis (meaning the curve bulges to the front of the neck), allowing our heads to sit on the top of our spine and look forward. This curve is a result of the discs being taller toward the front and shorter toward the back. Similarly, the lumbar spine has a natural lordosis, meaning the curve bulges toward the front as viewed from the side. The back muscles help pull the lumbar spine erect to position us upright; this creates the lumbar curve. Furthermore, in the lumbar spine, both vertebral bodies and discs are taller in the front.

The movements that can occur in the spine include forward bending (flexion), backward bending (extension), side bending (lateral flexion), and rotation. Twenty-four vertebrae comprise the spine and are divided into seven cervical, twelve thoracic, and five lumbar vertebrae (Figure 1). These are often written as cervical 1–7 (C1–C7), thoracic 1–12 (T1–T12), and lumbar 1–5 (L1–L5). The top of the sacrum is called sacral 1 (S1). The vertebral body can be divided two main regions, the vertebral body and the vertebral arch. The arch connects to the back of each body creating a space. This space is the spinal canal, in which the spinal cord is housed. The bone making up the body and arch is composed of a harder outer layer (called the compact or cortical bone), and a spongier inner core (called spongy or cancellous bone). Most of the spongy bone is in the core of the vertebral body and only a thin strip is found in the vertebral arch. On the very outside of the vertebral body there exists a tough tissue envelope called the periosteum, which is innervated by nerve endings and transmits pain sensation.

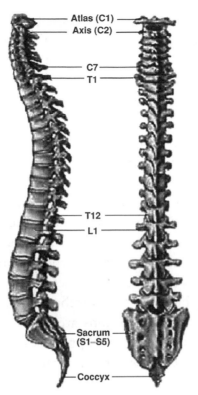

Atlas (C1)
Axis (C2)
C7
T1
T12
L1
Sacrum
(S1–S5)
Coccyx

Figure 1   Human spine from side and back views.

The vertebral body is the large anterior (toward the front) portion of the **vertebra** that acts to support the weight of the skull and body. These bodies are connected to each other by intervertebral discs made of cartilage. This creates a flexible pillar that can provide support to the human body, as well as protection to the spinal cord. Since more weight is borne by the vertebral bodies in the lower spine, as expected the vertebral bodies increase in size lower in the spine. The cervical vertebral bodies are the smallest, and the lumbar vertebral bodies are the largest.

The vertebral arch is made up of the pedicles and laminae. The pedicles are the rod-shaped parts that

Vertebra

one segment of the spine. The spine is comprised of seven cervical vertebrae, twelve thoracic vertebrae, and five lumbar vertebrae.

5

connect the arch to the back of the body, and the lamina is the part of the arch that makes the roof of the spinal canal. Also, ridges on the lamina are called spinous processes; these are the bumps that can be seen on the neck of a thin person who is looking down. When the vertebrae (with their body, pedicles, laminae, and spinous processes) stack on top of each other, they create holes on each side from which the spinal nerve roots can exit. These holes are called foramen, and the opening of the intervertebral foramen increases with forward bending (flexion) and decreases with backward bending (extension). As discussed previously, the vertebral bodies connect to each other through intervertebral discs. Similarly, there are connections between the vertebral arches, but rather than a **disc**, the connections are made through bony extensions called articular processes. The articular processes of neighboring vertebrae connect through joints called facets. The **facet** joint (like other joints) is made up of bone and cartilage. This joint receives significant sensory innervation.

Disc

the soft, gelatinous material that acts as a cushion between vertebrae in the spine. As we age, the disc degenerates or herniates and is often the source of back or neck pain.

Facet

the medical term for the spinal joint. Each vertebra has two facets, one on each site. The facets are often the source of pain for people with low back pain.

The last major structural components of the spine that are major contributors are the spinal ligaments. Ligaments connect bone to bone, and the spine has ligaments that extend along the entire front of the vertebral body (anterior longitudinal ligament), along the entire back of the vertebral body and on the front of the spinal canal (posterior longitudinal ligament), and along the back side of the spinal canal, just underneath the laminae (ligamentum flavum). Numerous other ligaments connect each body and facet to neighboring joints as well as the cervical spine to the base of the skull. See Figure 2.

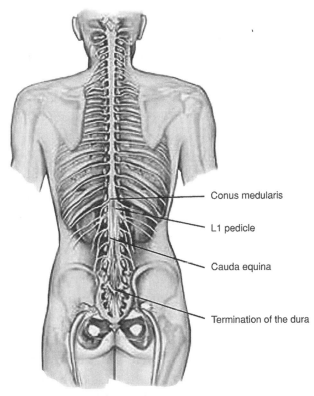

Conus medularis

L1 pedicle

Cauda equina

Termination of the dura

Figure 2   Spinal cord and spinal nerve roots.

2. What are the anatomy and function of the spinal cord and spinal roots?

The spinal cord is a cylindrical shaped structure that extends from the base of the skull down to the lumbar spine within the spinal canal. It is protected by the spinal column (within which it is encased), cerebrospinal fluid (within which it floats), and its outer tissue coverings called meninges (dura mater, arachnoid mater, and pia mater). The spinal cord and brain develop from the same embryological structure (the neural tube) and constitute the central nervous system (CNS). For the CNS to communicate with other structures in the body, such as muscles, blood vessels, and organs, it needs to receive and send electrical signals (called action potentials) via the peripheral nerves that constitute the peripheral nervous system (PNS). Within the context of this text the peripheral nerves that are most relevant are called spinal nerves. There are 31 pairs of spinal nerves attached to the spinal cord.

Spinal nerves primarily communicate with the neck, trunk, and extremities.

Spinal nerves primarily communicate with the neck, trunk, and extremities. When input is received by the spinal nerves, it is relayed to the spinal cord and integrated at the level of the spinal cord and sometimes modulated by signals from the brain. The response, which can be reflexive or voluntary, is returned to the periphery via the spinal nerve as well. Accordingly, the spinal nerve is a mixed nerve carrying both sensory and motor information. When the spinal nerve is at the level of the intervertebral foramen and within the spinal canal, it is actually split into its dorsal root (as it brings information into the spinal cord) and its ventral root (as motor signals are sent out of the spinal cord). The dorsal and ventral roots combine to form the spinal nerve at the intervertebral foramen. The spinal cord occupies only the upper two thirds of the spinal canal and in adults does not extend below the level of the second lumbar vertebral body. In children, the spinal cord extends lower.

The external features of the spinal cord represent its function. It is smooth with fissures and grooves (called sulci) and has dorsal and ventral roots attached to its side. The spinal cord is thicker in the cervical region and in the lumbar region, regions from where the spinal nerves responsible for the input and output to the extremities arise. The broadening at the end of the spinal cord in the upper lumbar region (L1 in adults) is called the conus medullaris. There are thirty-one spinal nerves: eight cervical (see Table 1), twelve thoracic, five

Table 1   Cervical roots

Nerve Root	C4	C5	C6	C7	C8
Muscle	—	Deltoid (lifts arms to the side)	Biceps (lifts hand to face)	Triceps (pulls hand away from face)	Hand muscles (moves fingers)
Sensation	Side of neck to bottom of head	Around shoulder and upper arm	Forearm and index finger	Forearm and middle finger	Forearm and little finger
Reflex		Biceps	Supinator	Triceps	

lumbar (see Table 2), five sacral, and one coccygeal. The lumbar spinal roots arise from the conus medullaris and are collectively called the *cauda equina* (Latin for horse's tail). Spinal roots exit the spinal column through the intervertebral foramen on each side.

The meninges of the spinal cord are worth discussing. The dura mater surrounds the spinal cord and spinal roots (up to the intervertebral foramen) from the base of the skull down to S2 (see Figure 3). Also, the pia

Table 2   Lumbar roots

Nerve Root	L3	L4	L5	S1
Muscle	—	Quadriceps (straightens leg)	Tibialis Anterior (lifts foot to allow standing on heal)	Gastrocnemius (allow) standing on (toes)
Sensation	Groin and inner thigh	Thigh	Top of the foot	Bottom of the foot
Reflex				Ankle

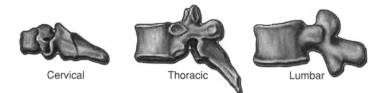

Cervical   Thoracic   Lumbar

Figure 3   Cervical, thoracic, and lumbar vertebrae.

mater has a thickened extension from the conus medullaris to the coccyx, called the filum terminale. This structure anchors the spinal cord to the inferior spine and is found within the lumbar spinal roots comprising the cauda equina.

The internal organization of the spinal cord is best observed in cross-section, demonstrating a distinct central H-shaped area of gray matter and a surrounding area of white matter. Also, within the center is a central canal that has a tiny amount of cerebrospinal fluid (CSF). The gray area is composed of nerve cell bodies. The white matter is composed of nerve cell extensions (called axons). Through these nerve cell bodies and axons, signals are relayed to and delivered from the brain. The information is transmitted within certain regions of the spinal cord called tracts. Motor information, sensory information, pain and temperature information, proprioception information (the ability to know spatial positioning of the body and extremities with your eyes closed), is carried in different tracts located in the spinal cord.

3. What are discs made of?

The intervertebral disc is essentially cartilage, made up of cells, water, and collagen. The structure is a dynamic one and has the capacity for degeneration with age and stress, with some limited capacity for repair. Because the disc has water, it can absorb load (which is what happens when we stand up or bend) by extruding water, and when the load is removed (when we lie down), the water returns to the disc from surrounding tissue and returns the disc height and volume. The disc has three anatomic regions: annulus (annulus fibrosus), nucleus (nucleus pulposus), and end plate. Each region has a distinct location (as described with their names) and distinct composition of fluid and cells. Accordingly, the functions of the three regions are different as well. The outer region of the discs is innervated and can generate pain.

The annulus surrounds the nucleus and is bound by the end plate above and below. The end plates are attached to the vertebral bodies. This structure provides support to the nucleus in the function of load bearing and is a relatively thick ring. The thinnest part of the annulus is at the sides in the back (posterolateral) of the disc. When disc herniations occur, they tend to occur in these areas. The annulus can also tear with stress; this is called an annular tear, making disc **herniation** through this area easier. Also, except for the outer region of the annulus, the disc is a structure without direct blood supply (avascular).

Herniation

condition that occurs when a material (usually a disc) squeezes out of its intended place. The herniated disc fragment often compresses an adjacent nerve or the spinal cord, causing pain or neurologic injury.

The nucleus is a rounded structure in the center of the intervertebral disc and is responsible for absorbing the fluid received by the disc from surrounding structures (a process called imbibition). As the nucleus ages or as the discs degenerate, the nucleus becomes less gelatinous, less able to extrude and absorb fluid with loading, and thereby less able to contribute to load-absorbing function in the spine. The disc also loses height from water loss (desiccation) with age and degeneration (see Figure 4).

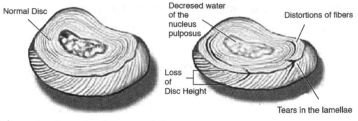

Figure 4   Normal and abnormal discs.

The end plate is essentially a pancake-shaped cap of the disc, above and below (superiorly and inferiorly), that attaches the disc to the vertebral body. Importantly, the end plate has holes (it is porous), allowing the disc to get nutrition from fluid entering and leaving the vertebral body. This structure, too, undergoes degeneration with age and stress.

4. What is the relationship of the spinal cord levels versus vertebral levels?

Spinal cord level is the portion of the spinal cord from which its respective pair of spinal roots arises. Because of unequal growth, the spinal cord resides only in the upper two thirds of the spinal column, and spinal cord levels don't necessarily correspond with vertebral levels. This is particularly true in the lumbar region where the lumbar spinal roots (and accordingly the spinal cord segment) arise more superior (above) than the level of the intervebral foramen from which it is intended to exit. For example, the L5 root arises from the conus but exits several vertebral levels below near the L5 vertebral body, or the L5 spinal cord level is not at the same level as the L5 vertebral level. In the cervical and thoracic spine, the spinal cord levels typically are at the level of their corresponding vertebral level. For example, the C7 spinal cord level is adjacent to the seventh cervical vertebral body.

5. What is the relationship of the spinal roots to the discs?

The spinal roots exit the spinal canal via the intervertebral foramen. The first seven spinal nerves (C1 to C7) exit above the body of the same number (for example, the C6 nerve exits the C6–C7 foramen)OK. Because there are only seven cervical vertebrae, but eight cervical nerves, the C8 nerve exits the C7–T1 foramen. From this nerve on to all the remaining thoracic and lumbar nerves below, each nerve exits below the vertebra of the same number (for example the L3 nerve exits the L3–L4 foramen) (Figure 5). This information is very important when the clinician evaluates what nerves will be compressed if a disc herniates. This varies with where in the spine the disc herniation occurs. A herniated disc in the neck (cervical disc herniation) will compress the nerve exiting below (for example, a disc herniation at C6–C7 will compress the C7 nerve). In the lumbar spine, the anatomy is different (because the spinal cord ends at L1–L2) but for reasons beyond the scope of this book, the nerve below will be compressed

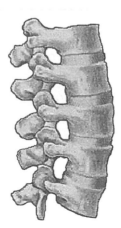

Figure 5   Normal spinal vertebrae and discs.

as well (for example, a disc herniation at L4–L5 will compress the L5 nerve root).

6. How does the spine develop?

The spinal column arises from tissue (mesoderm) adjacent to the neural tube (which gives rise to the brain and spinal cord—the CNS) during the embryological period. This tissue gives rise to cartilaginous areas that will eventually be turned into bone (ossified) and form the spinal column. The area that forms the vertebral body must fuse with the areas that lead to the posterior arch of the spinal column. This fusion happens during childhood.

Once someone is born, the spinal column continues to grow relative to the spinal cord. Thus, in babies the conus medullaris (the end of the spinal cord) is at the level of L2–L3. In adults it is usually at the level of L1. Thereby, injury to the spine, disc bulges, or invasive diagnostic procedures below the level of L2 in adults would not injure the spinal cord per se; however, lumbar spinal roots of the cauda equina would be vulnerable.

7. What happens to the spine as we age?

The spine has alternating segments that are fixed or mobile, and in the zones where these fixed and mobile segments transition into one another, mechanical stress is greatest. Accordingly, the lower cervical and the lumbar spine exhibit the most **degenerative** changes with time. As degeneration leads to bony formation at the disc and joints, movement becomes limited, and bony deposition can encroach upon the spinal canal and foramen. Additionally, degeneration can lead to changes in the spinal curves. The cervical and lumbar curves can lose their natural lordoses (the bulge toward

Degenerative

the changes that occur with normal aging. Degenerative diseases generally progress slowly.

front as viewed from the side), and become straight or even kyphotic (bulging toward the back as viewed from the side). This interferes with movement and load-bearing capacity, leading to further degenerative changes. See Figure 6 for an example of aged vertebrae.

The vertebral bodies change after the degeneration of the intervertebral discs. In order to help with increased stress of load bearing (since the discs are less effective), the bodies add bone to the areas immediately adjacent to the discs (called subchondral sclerosis). With accumulation of stress during a person's lifetime, the superior and inferior aspects of the vertebral bodies can generate new bone called osteophytes. These osteophytes tend to grow toward adjacent discs and in the cervical and lumbar spine toward the spinal canal as well. As degeneration progresses, the osteophytes and disc bulges narrow the opening of the foramen, and nerve roots are more likely to be compressed. This narrowing affects the width of the spinal canal as well.

In addition to osteophyte formation and intervertebral disc changes, all the other components of the spine can undergo degenerative changes as well. Joints can get

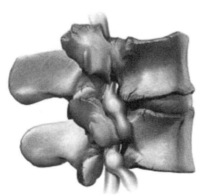

Figure 6   Aged vertebrae and disc with compression of nerve root.

larger (hypertrophy), ligaments can have bony deposi-
tions (ligamentous ossification), ligaments can grow
excessively (hypertrophy) and together comprise more
pathological changes that narrow the foramen for
nerve roots, narrow the canal for the spinal cord, and
limit the natural flexibility of the spine.

PART TWO

Degenerative Spine Disease— Discs

What is a herniated disc?

What can I do to help prevent degenerative spine disease?

What is the difference between radiculopathy and myelopathy?

More . . .

8. What is a herniated disc?

The nucleus of the intervertebral disc is contained within the annulus. When the nucleus squeezes into or out of the annulus, this is termed herniated disc. This herniation can occur after a sudden (acute) traumatic injury such as falling with bending of the neck, or, more commonly, it occurs after repetitive wear and tear lead to progressive thinning or fissuring of the annulus. The nucleus under load can escape into these fissures to the rim of the annulus and subsequent stress could lead the nucleus to actually extrude from the annulus into the spinal canal. Once in the disc space, it can impinge on a spinal nerve root, or in the cervical spine, the herniated disc can also impinge on the spinal cord. Since the nucleus is located slightly to the back (posteriorly) in the disc, and in the midline the annulus is bounded by the posterior longitudinal ligament, most disc herniations occur toward the back and side (posteriolaterally), the area where spinal roots are exiting the spinal canal through spinal foramen. Discs rarely herniate toward the front (anteriorly).

If the nucleus herniates up or down (superiorly or inferiorly) past the cartilaginous end plates into the verterbral body, it is called Schmorl's nodule. If the nucleus herniates into the annulus, causing the outer annular rings to bulge into the spinal canal, it is called disc protrusion. If the process continues, the nucleus may extend past the annulus into the spinal canal (but is still somewhat contained by the posterior longitudinal ligament), and it is called disc extrusion. Lastly, if the nucleus herniates past the annulus and posterior longitudinal ligament, so as to lie free in the spinal canal, it is called free fragment disc herniation.

Richard's comments:

The doctors weren't sure what caused my herniated disc. It definitely wasn't something I noticed immediately, the pain came on over a period of time. I did play sports, and did a bit of snowboarding, and I was told that these were probable causes.

9. What are the most common sites for degenerative spine disease?

The spine is constructed with alternating segments that are fixed and mobile. The transition between the segments is susceptible to the greatest wear and tear from mechanical stress. Accordingly, the cervical spine and the lumbar spine exhibit the greatest incidence of degenerative spine disease, which includes degenerative changes to the bone, ligaments, and discs.

In the cervical spine, more than 80% of disc herniations (see Figure 7) occur at C5–C6 or C6–C7, with the majority occurring at C6–C7. In the lumbar area, more than 90% of disc herniations occur at L4–L5 or L5–S1. The

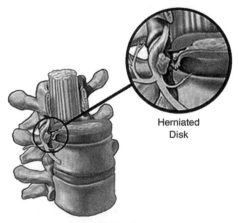

Herniated
Disk

Figure 7   Compression of nerve root by herniated disc.

bony aspects of the spine experience the greatest wear and tear at the joints (facet hypertrophy) as well as the osteophyte formation at the end plates and ligamentous calcification and overgrowth. Once again, these are local regions experiencing the most movement and stress.

10. What can I do to help prevent degenerative spine disease?

Degenerative changes in the spine are inevitable with increasing age (see Figure 8); however steps can be taken to minimize this degeneration as well as avoiding habits that may worsen it. First, any measure that reduces the load the spine needs to carry will lessen the speed with which the spine degenerates. Clearly, losing weight and being thin lessens the burden on the spine during standing as well as during bending. On the

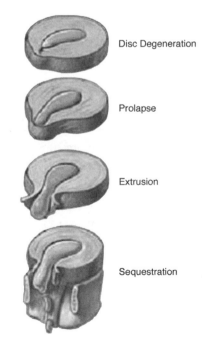

Disc Degeneration

Prolapse

Extrusion

Sequestration

Figure 8   Progression of herniated disc disease.

same note, strengthening the back muscles that are attached to the spine and serve to help with load sharing will reduce degenerative changes. Furthermore, thin people who exercise are less likely to injure their spine. Also very important is using techniques and body posture that do not place excessive strain on the spine. This includes maintaining a good posture in the workplace and using legs/hips to lift rather than bending. Lastly, smoking accelerates spine degeneration and slows recovery after spine injury or surgery.

11. What are the most common symptoms of herniated disc disease?

The symptoms of herniated discs vary with the region in which the disc has herniated. Cervical disc herniation can lead to compression of the spinal root or spinal cord. The symptoms a person may experience after disc herniation are related to what nerve is being compressed (see Table 3).

Table 3   Cervical disc herniation symptoms

Level of Disc Herniation	Root Compressed	Muscle Weakness	Distribution of Pain
C3–4	C4	No weakness in arm	Side of neck to bottom of head
C4–5	C5	Deltoid (lifts arms to the side)	Around shoulder and upper arm
C5–6	C6	Biceps (lifts hand to face)	Forearm and index finger
C6–7	C7	Triceps (pulls hand away from face)	Forearm and middle finger
C7–T1	C8	Hand muscles (moves fingers	Forearm and little finger

After cervical disc herniation, most patients will have some neck, shoulder, and/or arm pain, typically in a predictable pattern based on the nerve afflicted. The pain is usually sharp and radiating, and it may also have a dull, aching quality. Patients may also experience numbness and tingling in the arm and/or hand/fingers. Not uncommonly, patients with cervical disc herniation complain of headaches and may have some noticeable muscle wasting in the hands. If the cervical disc herniation is directed straight back, it may compress the spinal cord in the cervical spine. If this occurs, the patient may experience changes in the legs (clumsiness and/or dyscoordination in walking) as well as changes in bowel or bladder function.

Richard's comments:

I had progressive back pain that started as mere irritation, but it increased in severity and duration over time. I finally went to the doctor after my legs began going numb randomly because it became especially worrisome. By the time I was diagnosed I was also developing shooting pain down both my legs periodically.

Thoracic disc herniations, when occurring to the side, may cause pain in the nerve root that supplies the sensation to the skin over the ribs. However, since the thoracic nerve roots have little motor function, no weakness is usually detected. If the thoracic disc herniation is in the middle, it may compress the spinal cord and would lead to changes in the legs (clumsiness and/or dyscoordination in walking) as well as changes in bowel or bladder function.

Lumbar disc herniations (Table 4) occur predominantly in the lower lumbar regions (below L2), which is very important clinically. Since the spinal cord ends as

Degenerative Spine Disease—Discs

Table 4   Lumbar disc herniation symptoms

Level of Disc Herniation	Root Compressed	Muscle Weakness	Distribution of Pain
L2–3	L3	No weakness in arm	Side of neck to bottom of head
L3–4	L4	Deltoid (lifts arms to the side)	Around shoulder and upper arm
L4–5	L5	Biceps (lifts hand to face)	Forearm and index finger
L5–S1	S1	Triceps (pulls hand away from face)	Forearm and middle finger

the cauda equina at L1–L2, lumbar disc herniations cannot compress spinal cord. They can compress the respective nerve root, and if the herniation is large enough it may compress several nerve roots. Like in the cervical spine, the symptoms a patient would experience after lumbar disc herniation depend on which nerve root is being compressed. The typical patient will have lower back pain that radiates to the leg and/or foot. The pain is usually aggravated by movement, straining, or standing/sitting for an extended period of time. Often patients complain of muscle spasms in the lower back. The may also have weakness in the distribution of the affected nerve.

Patients often have several herniated discs and often present with disc disease in the cervical and lumbar region. In this scenario, it is critical to address the disc herniations that are causing the symptoms or endangering the spinal cord. Since cervical disc herniations into the spinal cord can lead changes in the legs, many surgeons will operate first in the neck with resolution of leg symptoms from relieving the compressive effects of cervical disc disease. Keep in mind leg pain doesn't arise from spinal cord compression and is usually a symptom of lumbar spinal root compression.

12. What is the treatment of a cervical herniated disc?

The treatment for a cervical herniated disc (Figure 9) can be nonoperative (conservative) or operative. For a great majority of patients who have cervical disc herniations, conservative therapy will be sufficient to improve their condition to relieve most of the pain and get them back to their activities of daily living. Conservative therapy includes bed rest, physical therapy, heat treatments, painkillers (analgesics), and muscle relaxants. It is reasonable to try conservative therapy for several weeks. Conservative management is for patients with pain and discomfort. If a patient has arm or hand weakness or signs/symptoms of spinal cord compression (clumsiness and/or dyscoordination walking, leg weakness, and any changes in bowel or bladder function), that patient should be evaluated immediately (usually with imaging and neurosurgical consultation).

Conservative management is for patients with pain and discomfort.

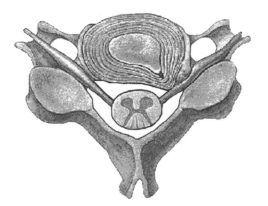

Figure 9   Compression of nerve root by cervical herniated disc.

25

If a patient has arm or hand weakness or signs/symptoms of spinal cord compression (clumsiness and/or dyscoordination walking, leg weakness, and any changes in bowel or bladder function), the patient should receive magnetic resonance imaging (**MRI**) of the cervical spine and be evaluated for a disc herniation that requires surgical **decompression**. Also, if a patient only has pain and continues to have severe pain after several weeks of attempted conservative therapy, the patient could be a candidate for surgical decompression if a herniated disc is diagnosed on imaging.

There are two main operations for the removal (decompression) of a herniated disc. The anterior cervical discectomy is performed through a 4-cm vertical incision on the side of the neck, and the incision can usually be hidden in a skin crease, leaving it undetectable in most patients several months after surgery. This incision allows access to the front (anterior) spine from which the disc can be removed with special surgical instruments and a microscope for enhanced illumination and magnification. Once the disc is removed, a small piece of bone is placed, which serves to build a bony connection between the vertebral body above and below (called spinal fusion). Lastly, a titanium plate with screws is placed on the front of the spine to help the fusion occur. Fusing two bodies in the neck has negligible consequences on the total range of motion of the cervical spine; the other cervical levels compensate well. This operation has a very high success rate. The other method of removing the herniated cervical disc is through a vertical incision on the back of the neck. This incision allows exposure of the back portion of the spine (lamina) from which a small hole can be drilled to remove the herniated disc. With this operation the

MRI

abbreviation for magnetic resonance imaging. A noninvasive diagnostic test that uses high-powered magnets to image parts of the body. This technique is very good at looking at soft tissues of the body, such as the spinal cord, discs, ligaments, and muscles.

Decompression

the removal of bone, disc, cartilage, ligament, or a tumor that is compressing on the spinal cord or nerve routes. Decompression surgery is often performed in conjunction with fusion if the amount of decompression is likely to cause spinal instability.

vertebral bodies are not fused, but not all cervical disc herniations can be removed from this approach.

13. What is the treatment of a herniated lumbar disc?

The treatment of a herniated lumbar disc can be nonoperative (conservative) or operative. For a great majority of patients who have lumbar disc herniations, conservative therapy will be sufficient to improve the patient's condition to relieve most of the pain and get them back to their activities of daily living. Conservative therapy includes bed rest, physical therapy, heat treatments, painkillers (analgesics), and muscle relaxants. It is reasonable to try conservative therapy for several weeks. Conservative management is for patients with pain and discomfort. If a patient has leg or foot weakness or signs/symptoms of bowel/bladder dysfunction, the patient requires immediate evaluation (usually with imaging and neurosurgical consultation).

Such a patient should receive magnetic resonance imaging (MRI) of the lumbar spine and be evaluated for a disc herniation that requires surgical decompression. Also, if a patient only has pain and continues to have severe pain after attempting conservative therapy for several weeks, this patient could be a candidate for surgical decompression if a herniated disc is diagnosed on imaging.

Lumbar disc herniations are usually treated with a lumbar discectomy via a vertical midline incision over the lower back. This incision allows exposure to the back of the lumbar spine (lamina) through which a small window can be drilled in the bone. This window almost always suffices to remove the lumbar disc herniation, and because of the architecture of the lumbar spine, the integrity and strength of the spine remains intact. Furthermore, a piece of bone is usually not necessary to be inserted in place of the removed lumbar disc.

14. What is a far lateral disc herniation?

To understand far lateral disc herniation it is worthwhile to review the relationship of the spinal roots to discs. The spinal roots exit the spinal canal via intervertebral foramen. The first seven spinal nerves (C1–C7) exit above the body of the same number (for example, the C6 nerve exits the C6–C7 foramen). Because there are only seven cervical vertebrae, but eight cervical nerves, the C8 nerve exits the C7–T1 foramen. From this nerve on to all the remaining thoracic and lumbar nerves below, the nerve exits below the vertebra of the same number (for example the L3 nerve exits the L3–L4 foramen). This information is very important when the clinician evaluates what nerves will be compressed if a disc herniates. This varies with where in the spine the disc herniation occurs. A herniated disc in the neck (cervical disc herniation) will compress the nerve exiting below (for example, a disc herniation at C6–C7 will compress the C7 nerve). In the lumbar spine, the anatomy is different (because the spinal cord ends at L1–L2) but for reasons beyond the scope of this book, the nerve below will be compressed as well (for example, a disc herniation at L4–L5 will compress the L5 nerve root).

Far lateral disc herniations happen most commonly the lumbar region. So a classical disc herniation in the lumbar region occurs toward the back and side (posteriolaterally), resulting in compression of the nerve root that is preparing to exit the level below (disc herniation at L4–L5 will compress the L5 nerve root). With a far lateral disc herniation, the direction of disc herniation is not toward the back and side (posteriolaterally), but directly to the side (laterally). With this the root that has already exited and classically not compressed is caught by the laterally herniating disc. So in a far lateral disc herniation, the L4–L5 disc herniation would compress and cause symptoms of the L4 root. This must be known before operating, as the operation would still involve a vertical midline incision, but the approach to the disc would more from the side of the spine versus a classic lumbar disc herniation.

15. What is the difference between radiculopathy and myelopathy?

The distinction between radiculopathy and myelopathy is very important to understand when considering the injury that can occur with herniated discs. Myelopathy is injury to the spinal cord. Since the spinal cord is in the cervical and thoracic spine, disc herniations into the spinal canal can compress the spinal cord, causing myelopathy. Myelopathy usually is not painful. It can cause symptoms at the level of injury and all levels below, such as numbness, weakness, dyscoordinated walking, clumsiness, and bowel or bladder changes. Lumbar disc herniations do not cause myelopathy because there are only lumbar roots in the spinal canal in the lumbar spine. So injuring the spinal cord and causing myelopathy only occurs with herniated discs at L1 or higher.

Radiculopathy is injury to the nerve root and can happen at any level of the spine, because nerve roots exit the spinal canal at each level of the spine. Radiculopathy is painful, usually sharp and radiating, but can have a dull aching component as well. Radiculopathy can also lead to numbness, tingling, and weakness in the distribution of the nerve affected. For example, a C5 radiculopathy could cause deltoid muscle weakness and pain radiating to the upper arm. Cervical disc herniations can cause both radiculopathy and myelopathy, sometimes called radiculomyelopathy.

16. What is cauda equina syndrome?

Cauda equina syndrome is an emergency.

Cauda equina syndrome is an emergency. Usually a herniated lumbar disc will compress only one or two roots and cause radiculopathy. If the disc herniation is massive, a large midline disc herniation can compress many lumbar roots leading to something called cauda equina syndrome. Patients will have significant weakness in the legs, not just in the distribution of one nerve root but in several major muscle groups. Severe back and leg pain is also common. Compressing multiple roots can also lead to bowel (fecal incontinence) and bladder changes (urinary retention or incontinence). Lastly, this syndrome is characterized by loss of sensation (anesthesia) in the anus and genitals region. This syndrome requires immediate evaluation with imaging, and usually surgical decompression to limit worsening of symptoms.

PART THREE

Degenerative Spine Disease— Stenosis and Spondylosis

What is OPLL?

What are the options for
decompressing spinal stenosis?

Are there risks to removing parts of the spinal column?

More ...

17. What is cervical spondylosis?

Spondylosis is another term for spine degeneration, more specifically spine degeneration that leads to the combination of disc height loss, bony (osteophyte) formation on the vertebral bodies, joint overgrowth (hypertrophy) and calcification and overgrowth of the ligaments (particularly ligamentum flavum). Together these changes are called spondylosis, which is wear and tear of the spine. These changes can lead to nerve root and/or spinal cord compression. So much like cervical disc herniation, cervical spondylosis can cause radiculopathy (compression of a nerve root), myelopathy (compression the spinal cord), or both.

Spondylosis
arthritis of the spine. It is associated with normal and abnormal motion of vertebrae over time.

When the above changes are present, the foramen and spinal canal are narrowed, so minor trauma can lead to significant injury. Patients may have chronic headaches, intermittent arm pain and weakness, some sensory loss, and neck pain. Unlike a single disc herniation that causes symptoms in the distribution of the nerve affected, cervical spondylosis can affect many roots. So the symptoms are more varied. Also, cervical spondylosis can occasionally cause altered blood flow to the brain (by compressing the vertebral artery that courses through the sides of the cervical vertebrae), and changes in swallowing have been reported from osteophytes pushing on the swallowing tube (esophagus).

Patients will usually be evaluated by plain X-ray and MRI, which reveal the classic features of cervical spondylosis. Then the clinician combines this information with the patient's history and physical examination to decide upon a therapeutic strategy. Conservative management, with bed rest, anti-inflammatory medicines, and physical therapy can help to some extent. If the patient has a very narrow canal (leaving little room for the spinal cord, especially if a trauma were to occur), worsening neurological changes, or out-of-control pain, surgical intervention is usually recommended.

The surgical options focus on decompressing the affected nerve roots and narrowed regions of the spinal canal. This can be achieved by an operation from the front of the neck or from the back of the neck. From the front, a small horizontal incision (in the crease of a wrinkle) is used to access the spine. Depending on the extent of the spondylosis, one to several vertebral bodies can be removed (corpectomy), with a bone strut or titanium cage (filled with bone) left in their place. The bone or cage will allow the bones to fuse over time, and the bony construct will turn into a long, stable segment of bone. Finally a plate and screws are placed in front of the bone strut or cage to hold things in place. From the back, a vertical incision is used to gain exposure to the back of the cervical spine. Then, using a drill, the surgeon removes the laminae over the compressed region, essentially unroofing the bone over the back of the spinal cord and relieving the compression.

18. What is OPLL?

OPLL stands for ossification of the posterior longitudinal ligament. This rare condition leads to significant bony deposition along the course of the posterior longitudinal ligament. The posterior longitudinal ligament runs up and down on the backside (posteriorly) of the vertebral bodies. This location is also the front side of the spinal canal, and thereby any overgrowth of the posterior longitudinal ligament can reduce the space available for the spinal cord within the spinal canal, leading to spinal cord compression. If this condition is diagnosed and the patient has symptoms, surgical decompression is indicated.

19. What is lumbar spinal stenosis?

Spinal **stenosis** is the narrowing of the spinal canal. This can occur from degeneration with time and stress (most often the case) or from a developmental condition that leads to a smaller spinal canal. This developmental spinal stenosis results from pedicles being too short, leading to a narrower spinal canal. For most, degeneration leads to bony spurs, joint overgrowth, and ligament overgrowth. Together these changes lead to spinal stenosis, which entraps the lumbosacral nerve roots in the constricted spinal canal and foramen.

The most characteristic complaints that people with lumbar spinal stenosis have are back and leg pain caused by standing and relieved by rest in a bent forward (flexed) or seated position. The pain can be sharp or dull and may involve both legs. Lumbar spinal stenosis is a chronic condition, and most people will have a degree of this as they age past 60 years. In fact, this condition is a very common cause of limited activity in the elderly and all the secondary negative consequences that result. A classic occurrence in people with lumbar spinal stenosis is that the pain gets better when they rest and when they bend forward. Bending forward results in flexion of the spinal canal and this opens the intervertebral foramen, freeing up the constricted lumbosacral nerve roots as they exit.

The diagnosis is most often made by clinical history. The patient can then be evaluated by plain X-rays and MRI to look more closely at each vertebral level.

Stenosis

narrowing of the spinal canal. It can occur gradually over time or acutely when a disc herniates or a vertebra fractures. If the narrowing is severe, then critical structures within the canal, such as nerves and the spinal cord, can be compressed, causing neurologic injury.

Degenerative Spine Disease—Stenosis and Spondylosis

35

Imaging reveals the classic narrowing of the spinal canal and foramen, with overgrowth of ligaments and facets. Disc bulges and height loss are common findings as well. The treatment begins with conservative therapy (unless the patient has weakness or bowel or bladder changes). If this fails after a reasonable period of time, surgery can be considered. The surgical procedures most often used are called lumbar laminectomy (removal of the laminae and unroofing the spinal canal, making more room toward the back for spinal cord) and foraminotomy (opening of the foramen, making more room for the exiting nerves). A vertical incision is made in the midline, and using a drill, the surgeon removes the laminae; subsequently, other instruments are used to open the foramen. Disc removal is usually not necessary. There are cases in which the pain is generated not only by the constriction of the spinal canal and foramen, but also by instability of the vertebral bodies. In this setting, the patient may need a lumbar fusion in which affected discs are removed and bone is inserted in their place to create a fusion between the adjacent vertebral bodies. Screws are inserted into the pedicles as well to securely hold the vertebral levels intended for fusion.

20. What is lateral recess syndrome?

When degenerative changes occur in the spine, some areas are particularly vulnerable to the growth of bony spurs and joints. When each lumbar nerve roots exits the cauda equina, it floats near the middle of the spinal canal. As the nerve prepares to exit its destined foramen, it takes a course toward the side of the spinal canal. The area of the spinal canal that is toward the side is called the lateral recess. This area borders the foramen and facets. With degeneration, the overgrown joints and bony spurs that have developed constrict the lateral recess. This can lead to nerve compression with even a small disc bulge, because the lateral recess is constricted in the degenerated spine.

21. Can spinal stenosis be confused with another diagnosis that is not caused by spine disease?

The most characteristic complaints that people with lumbar spinal stenosis have are back and leg pain caused by standing and relieved by rest in a bent forward (flexed) or seated position. The pain can be sharp or dull and may involve both legs. When a patient afflicted with lumbar spinal stenosis describes these symptoms, the condition is called neurogenic claudication. Neurogenic claudication is the progressive onset of radiating (radicular) leg pain, numbness, and in some cases weakness, that begins or is aggravated by walking. These people have increasing symptoms the more they walk. When they stop walking and sit down or bend forward, the symptoms are relieved within minutes. The symptoms do not get better for those who stop walking but stand straight up. This is because with bending forward, the foramen and spinal canal increase in size, relieving some of the compression on the nerve roots.

Neurogenic claudication needs to be differentiated from a different condition called vascular claudication (see Table 5), which does not arise from problems with the spine, but does cause leg pain that is relieved by rest. There are two conditions, one arising from spine disease (called neurogenic claudication) and the other arising from blood vessel disease (called vascular claudication), that can lead to leg pain with walking. Vascular

Table 5   Spinal stenosis versus vascular disease

	Spinal Stenosis	Vascular Disease
Symptoms	Neurogenic claudication	Vascular claudication
Pain started by	Walking	Walking
Pain relieved by	Rest (bending forward or sitting)	Rest (standing or sitting)
Pain caused by	Nerve compression	Low blood flow to leg muscles
Leg pulses	Normal	Decreased

Does the pain go away when you stop walking and remain standing? If it does, it is vascular claudication.

claudication results from insufficient blood flow to the leg muscles. The way to differentiate the two is by answering the following questions: Does the pain go away when you stop walking and remain standing? If it does, it is vascular claudication. Does the pain go away when you stop walking and remain standing? If it doesn't, it is most likely neurogenic claudication. Further confirmation can be gained if the person states that bending or sitting makes the leg pain go away.

22. What are the options for decompressing spinal stenosis?

The surgical procedure most often used for decompressing spinal stenosis is called lumbar laminectomy (removal of the laminae and unroofing the spinal canal, making more room toward the back for the spinal cord) and foramenotomy (opening of the foramen, making more room for the exiting nerves). A vertical incision is made in the skin directly over the midline and the back muscles are retracted to expose the back of the spine (laminae). Then, using a drill, the surgeon removes the laminae over the narrowed region. Before the operation, the surgeon identifies the region by studying the imaging and incorporating the patient's symptoms to the whole clinical picture. The bone is removed in the midline, and the facet joints off to the side are left undisturbed. Next, the surgeon uses other instruments to open the foramen (the holes from which the nerves exit) that are constricting spinal nerve roots. Disc removal is usually not necessary.

There are cases in which the pain is generated not only by the constriction of the spinal canal and foramen, but also by instability of the vertebral bodies. Back pain can arise from many sources including discs, joints, vertebral bodies, and nerve roots. So sometimes the best treatment is to take the motion out of the affected region by fusing it to the vertebral body above and to the vertebral body below. This is called spinal fusion, and although it takes away the motion (and thereby much or all of the pain that arises from the abnormal motion) across that part of the spine, the entire motion of the lumbar spine and spine as a whole is still retained. In a lumbar fusion, the affected discs are removed and bone is inserted in their place to create a fusion between the adjacent vertebral bodies. Screws are inserted into the pedicles as well to securely hold the vertebral levels intended for fusion.

23. What is spondylolisthesis?

Spondylolisthesis (Figure 10) is the slippage of a vertebral body forward so that body does not stack in line with the vertebral body below. Essentially, when one looks at the smooth lordotic (bulging forward) curvature of the spine, it is interrupted by one level having slid forward over the level below. This occurs because of a fracture in the lamina. Recalling the

Spondylolisthesis
a condition in which one vertebra slides out of position with respect to an adjacent vertebra. This most commonly occurs in the lumbar spine and is gradual and progressive in nature.

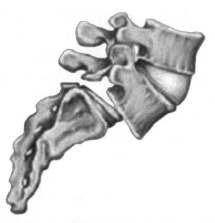

Figure 10   Spondylolisthesis (slipped vertebrae) of lower lumbar vertebra on sacrum.

anatomy of the spine, the laminae are connected to the vertebral bodies by the pedicles. Also, the laminae are connected to each other through the facet joints (this area of the laminae is called pars). A fracture of both joints or of the laminae connected to these joints would remove the posterior connection between the spinal segments. So at that affected level, the only connection that would keep the bodies from sliding forward would be the intervertebral disc. Accordingly, after a fracture of pars, the vertebral body at the fracture level can slide forward with time. When this occurs, it is called spondylolisthesis. If the L4 body has slid forward on the L5 body, it is called an L4/L5 spondylolisthesis.

This defect of fracture of the pars can occur as a stress fracture occurring over time or more suddenly (acutely) after trauma (see Table 6 for causes of spondylolisthesis). L5 is the most commonly affected level with spondylolisthesis, and L4 is the second most common. Spondylolisthesis can occur from other less common causes such as improper formation of the posterior spine

Table 6   Grading of spondylolisthesis

Grade	Amount of Slippage
I	<25%
II	25–50%
III	50–75%
IV	75% to complete

(called dysplastic type), breakdown of the facets, fracture of both pedicles, and bone diseases (Figure 11) affecting the posterior spine (Paget's disease). Spondylolisthesis is diagnosed by plain X-rays and computed tomography or computerized axial tomography (**CT** or **CAT** scan) or MRI imaging. After imaging, the degree of slippage is graded (see Table 7).

Spondylolisthesis can lead to back pain from the pathological movement of the bones and changes to the facet joints. Also, the slippage can compress spinal nerve roots, leading to leg pain and numbness.

CAT scan; CT scan abbreviations for computerized axial tomography (CAT) or computed tomography (CT) scan. A non-invasive diagnostic test that relies on X-rays and computerized reconstruction to image parts of the body. This technique is very quick and very good for looking at bone and dense instructions of the body.

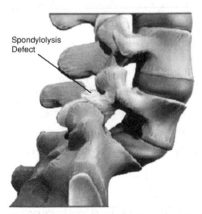

Spondylolysis Defect

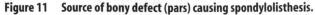

Figure 11   Source of bony defect (pars) causing spondylolisthesis.

Table 7 Causes of spondylolisthesis

Cause	Amount of Slippage
Isthmic	Fracture of pars Over time (stress) Suddenly (acute)
Degenerative	Intact pars, but facets erode with degeneration
Dysplastic	Congenital failure of posterior spine to completely form
Traumatic	Fracture of pedicles or facets
Pathological	Bone lesions that compromise the pars articularis

Carrie's comments:

I was born with spondylolisthesis, and my L5 had slipped 14 mm before it was diagnosed. I noticed that my outer calves and feet were constantly numb, and I would experience paralysis if I sat a certain way with my hips crooked, so I went to the doctors and they referred me to a neurosurgeon when they saw how far gone my spondylolisthesis was. The doctors were telling me that if the bone slipped any more, which can happen due to anything from slipping on the grass to a minor car accident, the paralysis would be permanent. So, it was crucial that I go under the knife.

24. How is spondylolisthesis treated?

It is important to know the grade and cause or spondylolisthesis prior to considering what is the best treatment. As with other spine diseases that are not causing instability in the spine, grade I or II spondylolisthesis can be treated with conservative management. Conservative therapy includes bed rest, physical therapy, heat treatments, painkillers (analgesics), and muscle relaxants.

It is reasonable to try conservative therapy for several weeks. Conservative management is for patients with pain and discomfort. If a patient has signs/symptoms of spinal cord compression (clumsiness and/or dyscoordination walking, leg weakness, and any changes in bowel or bladder function), this patient should be evaluated immediately (usually with imaging and neurosurgical consultation). For people who have a higher grade spondylolisthesis (grade III and IV), a surgeon should be consulted to see if spinal decompression and/or spinal fusion is indicated. This condition can cause both spinal nerve compression and spinal instability. Also, in certain patients, the vertebral bodies need to be restacked (reduced) before fusion, whereas if the slippage is minimal the fusion can be performed without restacking.

Carrie's comments:

My spondylolisthesis had progressed quite a bit before I was diagnosed, and I was told I had higher grade spondylolisthesis (14 mm slippage of the L5) that needed to be treated with a spinal decompression and fusion between L5 and S1 because of compression of the spinal cord and possible permanent paralysis if any further slippage occurred. The thought of having my back cut open and my spine fused together was definitely very alarming. The news began a very harrowing process of preparing for surgery, going through the operation, and recovering.

25. What is basilar invagination?

The anatomy of the cervical spine as it connects to the base of the skull is unique and is collectively called the craniovertebral junction. The base of the skull has a hole (foramen magnum) from which the brain stem exits and turns into the spinal cord. Surrounding the

Occipital

a term used to refer to the back and bottom part of the skull. This is the part of the skull that is in contact with the top of the spine.

foramen magnum are two smooth surfaces on the bottom of the skull called **occipital** condyles. It is these surfaces that rest the skull on the first vertebra of the cervical spine. The first vertebra is called the atlas. Much of the head's ability to move down and up (flexion and extension) occurs at this joint. The first vertebra rests on the second vertebra, which is called the axis. This joint is different from all other spinal levels. The second vertebra has a fingerlike bony projection that extends upward and attaches to the inside front part (anterior) of the first vertebra. This bony extension is called the dens. This joint between the first and second vertebra provides a significant contribution to the ability of the head to turn from side to side (rotation).

The diseases that can occur at the craniovertebral junction include the fusion of the first vertebra to the base of the skull. When this occurs, sometimes the base of the skull can settle down into the spine, leading to the ascension or upward extension of the second vertebra into the foramen magnum. Since the second vertebra has the dens, this can ascend into the foramen magnum and compress the bottom portion of the brain stem just prior to its transition into the cervical spinal cord. This is called basilar invagination or basilar impression. The entire disease process ultimately leads to the settling of the spine into the base of the skull, which can even reduce the volume of the back portion of the skull, which houses a part of the brain called the cerebellum.

Congenital

a disease that came prior to birth. This is opposed to degenerative, which occurs as one ages.

Basilar invagination occurs in **congenital** conditions (Down syndrome, Flippel-Feil syndrome, and Chiari malformation) that have a higher rate of abnormalities in the craniocervical junction. It can also occur from acquired conditions (rheumatoid **arthritis**, as shown in Figure 12, or trauma). Patients who have basilar invagination can have problems involving the function of the lower brain stem. Patients can have respiratory and balance problems (from cerebellum compression) as well as problems with swallowing and speaking (functions of cranial nerves that originate from the lower brain stem).

The treatment depends on the degree of spinal canal reduction and compression of spinal cord or brain stem. The compression is usually from the upward-driven dens of the cervical vertebra. Patients who need surgery will need a decompression (to make space for the spinal cord or brain stem) and fusion of the craniocervical junction (to keep the bones from settling any further). Decompression can be achieved by removing the dens during an operation through the mouth or from removal of the laminae from behind. Fusion requires placing screws and rods securely linking the base of the skull, first vertebra, and second vertebra.

Arthritis

normal aging and wear and tear on bones and joints causes inflammation and pain referred to as arthritis. This can occur at any joint in the body and is common in the joints of the neck and low back.

Degenerative Spine Disease—Stenosis and Spondylosis

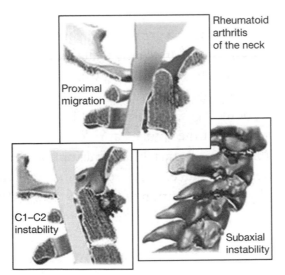

Rheumatoid arthritis of the neck

Proximal migration

C1–C2 instability

Subaxial instability

Figure 12   Effects of rheumatoid arthritis on the cervical spine.

26. Are there risks to removing parts of the spinal column?

The spine is both very stable and very flexible. This flexibility is maintained through the interactions of ligaments, discs, joints, and muscle. Accordingly, many operations that remove tissue or bone and still leave the spine as a mechanical device structurally intact can be performed. For example, the removal of laminae in the posterior cervical spine for cervical spondylosis is done so the joints are left intact. This opens the spinal canal but doesn't make the spine unstable. Unfortunately, it may make the spine more likely to take on an unnatural curve over time, so this can be addressed by leaving in screws and rods to resist this gradual deformation.

If discs are removed from the cervical spine, they can be substituted with bone.

Sometimes, removed parts can be replaced. If discs are removed from the cervical spine, they can be substituted with bone. This allows the vertebra above and below to join each other through the bone that has been inserted in the evacuated disc space. In the lumbar spine, however, during a lumbar discectomy the disc can be removed without the need to replace it; this does not compromising the integrity of the spine. Understanding the architecture and design allows the surgeon to decide whether the spine is highly unstable or at risk of slowly developing deformation. If the spine is highly unstable, bony cages, screws, and rods can be placed to create stability. If the spine is at risk of slowly developing deformation or instability, the options could include wearing a brace. However, the best treatment is created by internal fixation with screws and rods.

PART FOUR

Spine Trauma

What is a burst fracture?

Which fractures can be treated with a brace?

How long does it take for a fracture to heal?

More ...

27. What are osteoporosis and osteopenia?

Like other tissue in the human body, bone is continuously being absorbed and deposited in a balance that maintains the strength of the bone. This balance is mediated by osteoblasts (which add bone cells) and osteoclasts (which remove bone cells), and if too much bone is removed by osteoclasts or not enough bone is added by osteoblasts, bone can become weak and more likely to break. People with **osteoporosis** most often break bones in the hip, spine, and wrist. The definition of osteoporosis is either a bone mineral density (BMD) 2.5 standard deviations below peak bone mass as measured by dual energy X-ray absorptiometry (DXA), or any fragility fracture. The definition of **osteopenia** is bone density that is lower than normal but not low enough to be called osteoporosis. Based on the BMD as evaluated by DXA, a T-score is given. A T-score > 1 is normal, a T-score between 1 and 2.5 is considered to be low and sometimes termed osteopenia, and a T-score above 2.5 is considered diagnostic of osteoporosis.

Osteoporosis can lead to osteoporotic fractures (see Figure 13), which are fractures that occur under little stress that typically wouldn't lead to a fracture in a nonosteoporotic person. The vertebra column is a common site for osteoporotic fracture. The risk factors are important to discuss because prevention remains the better strategy over treatment when it comes to osteoporosis.

The diagnosis of osteoporosis is made by DXA, which evaluates the patient's BMD, but it is important to remember that a fracture from low level trauma (most likely osteoporotic fracture) is also di-

Osteoporosis

a bone condition in which bone mineral density is reduced substantially and bone collagen is disrupted. Bones become weaker and people with the condition are at higher risk of developing a fracture.

Osteopenia

a decrease in bone mineral density that occurs in some people as they age. It can be a precursor to osteoporosis, though not everyone with osteopenia develops osteoporosis.

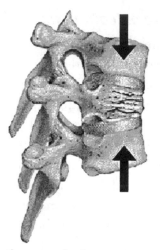

Figure 13 Osteoporotic compression fracture.

agnostic of osteoporosis regardless of the findings on DXA. As mentioned previously, prevention is the key, and if a patient is diagnosed with osteoporosis, there are several medicines that can help maintain and add bone density. The vertebrae have trabecular bone in the central part that is constantly remodeling; if this balance is altered and the bone density decreases, the patient is at risk for a vertebral fracture (see Table 8 for risk factors for osteoporosis). Furthermore, if surgical management is necessary, the results are less favorable when patients have bone that is osteoporotic.

28. What is a compression fracture?

A compression fracture of the spinal vertebrae is one in which the front (anterior) end of the vertebral body is compressed. Importantly, the back (posterior) part of the vertebral body maintains a normal height when compared to adjacent vertebral bodies. This type of

Table 8 Risk factors for osteoporosis

Non-Modifiable	Potentially Modifiable
• History of a fracture	• Prolonged steroid use
• Female sex	• Tobacco smoking
• Advanced age	• Estrogen deficiency
• Dementia	• Menopause before 45 years of age
• European or Asian background	• Alcoholism
	• Sedentary lifestyle
	• Certain intestinal diseases

fracture is also sometimes called a wedge fracture, because as viewed from the side the vertebral body, the vertebra changes from its typical columnar shape to the appearance of a wedge.

Wedge fractures (Figure 14) can occur during trauma that leads to compression of the spine while the spine is

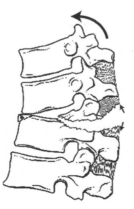

Figure 14   Wedging and forward bending of the spine as a result of a fracture.

51

A burst fracture is caused by compression of the spine while it is in the neutral position, meaning not flexed or extended. A burst fracture usually occurs after significant trauma. This compressive force leads to height loss of the entire vertebral body as well as extension of some collapsed bone into the spinal canal. This can lead to injury of the spinal cord and or roots depending on the level where the burst fracture occurs. The diagnosis is made by X-rays and CT scan.

A burst fracture is unstable and will need either a brace or surgery. If the burst vertebra has maintained most of its height, and if there is no collapsed bone extending into the spinal canal, the patient may be a candidate for a brace. If there is significant height loss, or forward bending of the entire spine as a result of this fracture (called kyphosis) or significant extension of bone into the spinal canal, most likely the patient will need surgery. The decision depends on many other factors about the patient's health and is made with the entire clinical scenario in mind.

30. What is an odontoid fracture?

The odontoid is part of the C2 vertebra and an odontoid fracture is accordingly a fracture of the C2 vertebra. This vertebra is unique from all other spinal vertebrae in that it has a bony prominence that extends upwards (cephalad) from the front (anterior) part of the C2 vertebra. This upward part of the C2 vertebra is called the odontoid, and it connects with the C1 vertebra (the C1 vertebra is more like a ring and doesn't have the typical thick vertebral body). By connecting to C1, the odontoid serves as pivot around which C1 and the skull can rotate. In fact, 50% of the rotation (ability to look from side to side) we have in our necks is from the odontoid of C2 connecting to C1. Because this area is more flexible than other spinal levels, it is also susceptible to fracture. Such a fracture is called an odontoid fracture. Depending on where the fracture line is, odontoid fractures can be classified as Type I through Type III (see Table 9).

Patients who have odontoid fractures commonly report a fall or trauma with their necks bent forward during the event. This usually leads to neck pain and stiffness, and if it is severe, patients may even have weakness and numbness in the arms or legs. Diagnosis is made by X-rays and can be further evaluated by CT scan.

The two most common types are Type II (Figure 17) and Type III (Figure 18). Type III fractures are considered to be unstable, meaning some intervention must be taken to help the fracture heal. For Type III fractures, this can be achieved with a neck brace that prevents motion in the neck region, allowing the fracture to heal. For Type II fractures, many times a brace is insufficient and surgery with the placement of a single screw through the C2 vertebra and the odontoid needs to be performed. On occasion, the screws will need to be placed from the back of the neck to join C1 and C2 so the fractured odontoid doesn't lead to spinal cord injury.

Table 9   Types of odontoid fractures

Type I	Type II	Type III
• Fractured through tip, stable	• Fractured through base of neck, unstable	• Fractured through body of C2, stable

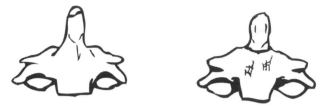

Figure 17   **Fracture through neck of odontoid (Type I & II odontoid fracture).**

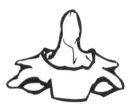

Figure 18   **Fracture through body of C2 (Type III odontoid fracture).**

31. What is a hangman's fracture?

One type of fracture is named hangman's because when someone is hanged, this vertebra is the one that is broken by the knot of the noose. More commonly, this fracture occurs when there is compressive force on the head while the neck is extended (when one bends one's neck to look up, the neck is extended). The forces lead to a fracture of C2 vertebra in the area of the pedicles (the bony parts that connect the body of the vertebra to the lamina and form the lateral aspects of the spinal canal). The C2 vertebra can be fractured at the odontoid or the pedicles, which is a hangman's fracture.

Patients who have a hangman's fracture commonly report a fall or trauma with their necks bent backward during the event. This usually leads to neck pain and stiffness, and if the case is severe, patients may even have weakness and numbness in the arms or legs. Diagnosis is made by X-rays and can be further evaluated by CT scan.

The fracture is evaluated by imaging to define several important characteristics such as how bent (angulated) or misaligned (subluxed) the disrupted spinal level is. Based on these characteristics, the surgeon may recommend traction, bracing, and/or surgery.

32. What is a Jefferson's fracture?

A Jefferson fracture is a fracture of C1 which typically happens during car accidents with compressive force on the top of the head with the neck in neutral position. The force is spread out over the ring shape of C1 and leads to fractures that break the ring. Usually the pieces fall outward and away from the canal. Because of the fracture pattern and anatomy, the spinal cord is rarely injured.

Patients who have a Jefferson's fracture commonly report a fall or trauma with their necks straight during the event. This usually leads to neck pain and stiffness, and if it is severe, the patients may even have weakness and numbness in the arms or legs. Diagnosis is made by X-rays and can be further evaluated by CT scan.

The majority of Jefferson's fractures can be treated with a brace that prevents movement in the cervical spine, allowing for the fracture to heal. On occasion, a patient may need surgery, especially if the fracture is associated with other fractures in the neck.

33. What is vertebra dislocation?

A dislocated vertebra is a severe injury which usually happens after a severe trauma. In order to understand what occurs when a vertebra is dislocated, a review of spinal anatomy and connections is necessary. The vertebral body is the large anterior (toward the front) portion of the vertebra I think this spelling is ok, vertebra is singular and vertebrae is plural. that acts to support the weight of the skull and body. These bodies are connected to each other by intervertebral discs made of cartilage. This creates a flexible pillar that can provide support to the human body as well as protection to the spinal cord. As discussed previously, the vertebral bodies connect to each other through intervertebral discs. Similarly, there are connections between the vertebral arches, but rather than a disc, the connections are made through bony extensions called articular processes. The articular processes of neighboring vertebrae connect through joints called facets. The facet joint (like other joints) is made up of bone and cartilage. This joint receives significant sensory innervation. The last major structural components of the spine that are major contributors are the spinal ligaments. Ligaments connect bone to bone, and the spine has ligaments that extend along the entire front of the vertebral body (anterior longitudinal ligament), along the entire back of the vertebral body, on the front of the spinal canal (posterior longitudinal ligament), and along the back side of the spinal canal, just underneath the laminae (ligamentum flavum). Numerous other ligaments connect each body and facet to neighboring joints as well as the cervical spine to the base of the skull.

In order to dislocate a vertebral body, the traumatic forces must disrupt the discs that connect the vertebral bodies or fracture though the entire spinal level, including the vertebral body and lamina, and/or fracture the joints that link the levels. This leads to a grossly unstable spine that needs surgical intervention to create stability.

As expected, this type of injury is often associated with damage to the spinal cord or spinal roots. When evaluation is performed with X-rays and CT scan, the dislocated vertebra leads to a step-off where the lines and curves of the spinal column are no longer smooth.

34. What are transverse or spinous process fractures?

Not all fractures of the spinal column or vertebrae are clinically important. The spinous process and transverse process of the vertebrae are bony projections that can be fractured without any clinical consequence and do not need to be treated. The spinous process is the bony process you can feel on the back of your neck when you look down. It extends from the middle of the lamina and is the site of muscular attachments. However, a fracture of the spinous process does not need to be treated and will heal sufficiently on its own. Similarly, the transverse processes are the projections that extend from the side of the vertebral body and pedicles. These are also used for muscular attachments and don't need to be treated for sufficient healing. The discovery of a spinous or transverse process fracture raises the concern for a clinically significant fracture elsewhere in the spine and will lead the clinician to look at the entire spine more closely.

The discovery of a spinous or transverse process fracture raises the concern for a clinically significant fracture elsewhere in the spine and will lead the clinician to look at the entire spine more closely.

35. What is occipital dislocation?

Also known as craniocervical disruption, an occipital dislocation is very uncommon, comprising less than 1% of cervical spine injuries. This type of injury is from a very severe traumatic force, and most patients present with neurological deficit or death from stretching of the spinal cord and brain stem (bulbar-cervical dissoci-

Spine Trauma

ation). The treatment is occipitocervical fusion, which uses screws and rods to reattach the base of the skull to the top of the spine.

36. Does a spine fracture always lead to weakness or paralysis?

No, a spine fracture does not always lead to weakness or paralysis. Fractures can lead to weakness or paralysis if the nerve roots or spinal cord are compressed even for a short period of time. Also, if a fracture leads to no neurological injury when the fracture happens, it may still cause injury to the nerve roots and spinal cord if the spinal column becomes unstable and collapses over time. Spinous process and transverse process fractures typically don't cause any neurological deficit, and occipital dislocation or vertebral dislocation typically do cause some amount of weakness or paralysis. Many other fractures fall somewhere in between and depend on the fracture pattern and other more subtle factors.

After a fracture, if the spine is left unstable without stabilization (whether by brace or surgery), the fracture can serve as a point for further collapse or further alteration of the natural spinal curvature. This can lead to what is called spinal deformity, which can lead to compression of nerve roots or the spinal cord.

37. Which fractures can be treated with a brace?

Some fractures that leave the spine unstable can be treated with a brace, allowing the fracture to heal and leaving the spine structurally stable after that healing process has occurred. This is only possible for fractures that have been studied over time to be treatable with a

Table 10   Fractures that *may* be treatable with a brace

Location in Spine	Fracture
Cervical	• Jefferson's • Odontoid • Hangman • Wedge
Thoracic	• Wedge • Burst
Lumbar	• Wedge • Burst

Spine Trauma

brace (see Table 10). Typically these fractures do not have a significant amount of height loss or bending (angulation) of the spine and do not have bony fragments in the spinal canal that may need surgical removal.

Essentially what a brace does is allow the fractured area to remain still while the natural mechanisms of bone healing are under way. If there is motion over or through the fractured area, bone healing fusion will not occur and the fracture will remain. Similarly, in surgery, the rods and screws are used provide a motion-free environment for healing to occur, but with surgery, additional bone can be added so the healing occurs and re-creates the normal shape and curvature of the spine.

38. Which fractures need surgery to stabilize?

Some fractures that leave the spine unstable can only be treated with surgery (Table 11), allowing the frac-

Table 11   Fractures that may be treated with surgery

Location in Spine	Fracture
Cervical	• Occipital dislocation • Jefferson's • Odontoid • Hangman • Burst • Vertebra dislocation
Thoracic	• Burst • Vertebra dislocation
Lumbar	• Burst • Vertebra dislocation

ture to heal and leaving the spine structurally stable after that healing process (Figure 19). With surgery, many types of correction are possible, including restoring height to collapsed vertebrae, restoring the normal curvature, and removing bony fragments that may be compressing spinal nerves or spinal cord.

Essentially, screws are used to grab (acquire) parts of the vertebrae and are connected to rods that allow the fractured area to remain still while the natural mechanisms of bone healing are under way. If there is motion over or through the fractured area, bone healing fusion will not occur and the fracture will remain. Additionally, the abnormal curvature of the spine after some fractures can be corrected during surgery and maintained with the **instrumentation** used (scews, rods, and wires). Furthermore, ground-up bone in titanium cages with substances that promote bone growth can be inserted where the fracture leaves vertebrae completely destroyed and insufficient for proper healing.

Instrumentation

The placement of foreign material used to fuse or aid in the structure of the spine. Most instrumentation involves titanium rods and screws that are implanted in the spine and hold it in proper position while healing or arthrodesis occurs.

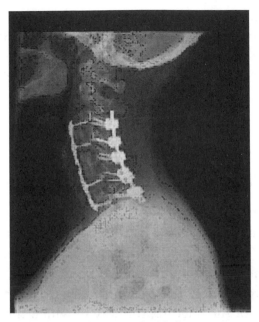

Figure 19   Lateral X-ray of spine after spinal fusion surgery.

39. What is a halo orthosis?

There are many different types of braces designed specifically for each of the various types of fractures as well as the various regions of the spine in which they occur. Typically, the thoracic and lumbar spine braces are hard shelled and form fitted (after measurement and custom design), resembling a sort of turtle shell. A halo orthosis a brace designed to stabilize the upper cervical spine, and for fractures of the C1–C3 vertebrae. It is called a halo because part of the brace is fitted around the shoulders and upper chest and has prominent metal rod extensions that are connected to a metal ring (hence the term halo). For the chest and shoulder part of the brace to be connected securely to the head, and thereby not allowing any movement of the neck, it has to be connected to the metal halo ring that is fixed to the

Spine Trauma

63

skull. The ring has screws that are fitted into the outer part of the skull at four different points under local anesthesia. This is done at the bedside, and afterwards the patient is only responsible for keeping the screw sites clean. The halo orthosis and surgery are the usual treatment options for patients with C1 or C2 fractures.

40. How long does it take for a fracture to heal?

The time it takes for a fracture to heal depends upon several criteria. Specifically, it is determined by the location of the fracture in the vertebra, the location of the vertebra in the spine, the age of the patient, the severity of the fracture, the way in which the fracture was treated, and other medical conditions from which the patient may suffer (osteoporosis, diabetes, etc.).

Body casts are not used any more.

Fortunately, most fractures of the spine are not comminuted. This means that the bone fragments are in close proximity to one another. In this situation, fractures can heal in as quickly as 6 weeks in healthy individuals if the vertebra is immobilized. Immobilization can be achieved through surgery or external bracing. Body casts are not used any more. Comminuted fractures are generally more severe and often require surgery. The fractures can take longer to heal (up to three months). On occasion, a vertebra is fractured so severely that it cannot be salvaged, and the fragments need to be removed and the spine reconstructed with titanium cages, rods, and screws. In this case, 2 or more vertebrae are fused together. The time it takes for fusion to become solid can take as long as 12 months, although evidence of fusion is usually noticed within 6 months.

Older patients, smokers, and those with certain types of fractures (e.g., Type II odontoid fractures) are at higher risk of having a fracture never heal. This is referred to as a nonunion. A nonunion may be a source of persistent pain and instability and is often an indication for surgery.

PART FIVE

Spinal Cord Injury

What is a spinal cord injury?

What are the prognosis and long-term management of spinal cord injury?

What resources are available to me if I suffered a spinal cord injury?

More . . .

41. What is a spinal cord injury?

Spinal cord injury (SCI) refers to damage (temporary or permanent) to the spinal cord itself, which may or may not be associated with fractures of the spinal column. The damage has consequences to the patient that depend on where the spinal cord is injured and the type and severity of spinal cord injury.

Roughly 250,000 spinal injuries occur in the United States each year and approximately 10% are associated with severe neurological injury, with 0.5% resulting in death. The overwhelming majority of traumatic spinal cord injuries involve the cervical region of the spine since it is the most mobile portion. The majority of cervical spine injuries occur in patients 18 to 30 years old and are most commonly associated with motor vehicle accidents (including motorcycle accidents). In comparison with the injuries in younger populations, spinal cord injuries of patients over 65 years of age are more commonly associated with falls. See Table 12 for common causes of spinal cord injuries. SCI after spine trauma depends on the type and level of injury, the force associated with the trauma, the age of the patient, and the patient's general health prior to the injury. Most patients who suffer a cervical spine fracture may also have injuries to other organs that can cause shock and hypoxia, which can exacerbate spinal cord damage.

Table 12   Causes of spinal cord injury

Motor vehicle accident (50%)
Fall (20%)
Sports (15%)
Violence (10%)
Other (5%)

Spinal Cord Injury

In order to understand the SCI, a review of the spinal cord anatomy is necessary. The spinal cord extends from the bottom of the skull to the upper lumbar spine. There are two swellings in the shape of the cord in the cervical and lumbar regions that correspond to the origin of the spinal roots to the arms and legs, respectively. Cerebrospinal fluid bathes the cord and can be easily sampled by a needle in the lower back with a spinal tap (lumbar puncture). The bony spinal column provides protection to the spinal cord as well as support and flexibility to the trunk.

Damage to the spinal cord can affect the various tracts of neurons carrying sensory and motor information back and forth between the brain and the body. Depending on the location of the SCI patients can have distinct combinations of motor or sensory loss. Also, the brain's control over the bladder and bowels is altered, leading to inability to void and defecate.

42. What are the different types of SCI?

When a patient suffers from trauma and there is concern that the spinal cord may be injured, it is the examination of the patient's motor and sensory function that reveals what type of SCI has occurred. This assessment is made again after 24 hours to establish the final diagnosis. SCI is categorized by two critical features. The first feature is the highest level of the spinal cord that is injured (whether the injury is in the neck, the thoracic spine, or the upper lumbar spine), which will dictate how much loss of function the patient suffers. The second feature is the completion of the injury—the patient can have either a complete (no function below the level of injury) or incomplete (some function below the level of injury) spinal cord injury (see Table 13). Further, incomplete spinal cord injury has different varieties (Figure 20) that lead to unique combinations of motor and sensory loss (see Table 14).

Table 13 Types of spinal cord injury

Complete Spinal Cord Injury	Incomplete Spinal Cord Injury
• Complete loss of voluntary movement, bladder control, and sensation below the level of the injury • No preservation of motor and sensory function below injury level • The persistence of a complete spinal cord injury beyond 24 hours indicates that no function will recover • Low blood pressure, slow heart rate	• Some motor and sensory function persists below level of injury • Central Cord Syndrome • Anterior Cord Syndrome • Brown-Sequard Syndrome

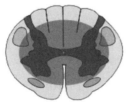

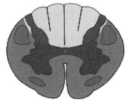

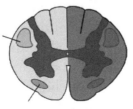

Figure 20   Central cord syndrome (top), anterior spinal artery syndrome (middle), and Brown Séquard syndrome (bottom).

Table 14   Types of incomplete spinal cord injury

Central Cord Syndrome	Anterior Cord Syndrome	Brown-Sequard Syndrome
• Most common type of incomplete spinal cord syndrome • Arm weakness prominent, some leg weakness • Surgery often performed on a non-urgent basis	• Usually from low blood flow in the spinal artery • Motor deficit and loss of pain and temperature sensation • Preservation of some sensation	• Spinal cord injured to the middle without injury to the other half of the spinal cord • Usually due to penetrating trauma • Loss of motor function of same side of injury • Loss of pain and temperature sensation on opposite side of injury

43. How is a spinal cord injury treated when it occurs?

When a person is involved in a traumatic event, great concern is given to evaluate for SCI. Patients are kept on a rigid board while they are screened for SCI with physical examination and imaging evaluation. Plain X-rays are helpful as a screening imaging test. CT scan is the imaging study of choice to diagnose fracture/dislocation. MRI is the imaging study of choice to diagnose spinal cord injury, disc herniation, and ligamentous injury. SCI is usually seen as a bright signal in the substance of the cord that occurs from postinjury edema.

Some patients who suffer a spinal cord injury are neurologically devastated at the time of the initial impact, generally as a result of spinal cord transection. These patients will have SCI that does not improve despite aggressive treatment of low blood pressure, low blood oxygenation, and spinal fractures. This type of injury is referred to as complete spinal cord injury. Less devastating injuries are commonly referred to as incomplete spinal cord injury and have the potential for neurological recovery, a potential maximized by aggressive treatment of low blood pressure, low blood oxygenation, and spinal fractures.

In addition, the early administration of steroids, specifically methylprednisolone, immediately (best if administered within 8 hours of injury) after severe spinal cord injury can increase the likelihood of subsequent neurological recovery. Scientific investigation has shown that after the actual injury of the spinal cord, events are begun that further the injury, particularly the initiation of the inflammatory process; this inflammatory damage can be minimized with steroids (potent anti-inflammatory agents). While being treated with a steroid regimen, patients will be placed on gastrointestinal protective agent medicines to prevent the formation of stomach ulcers (a known complication of steroid use).

44. What are the prognosis and long-term management of spinal cord injury?

The prognosis of SCI and the long-term management are highly dependent on each other, and they are also very dependent on the level of paralysis. If a person has a cervical spinal cord injury and cannot move his arms or legs, he is referred to as quadriplegic. If the injury is below the cervical spinal cord and the function of the arms is retained, while leg function and trunk muscle function is lost, he is referred to as paraplegic. The prognosis and long-term management of quadriplegics and paraplegics is different.

Quadriplegic patients are further classified as either ventilator dependent or independent. Based on the anatomy of the cervical spinal cord, the nerves that control the breathing (diaphragm muscle) arise from cervical 3–4–5 segments. Any injury to these levels will leave the patient ventilator dependent. These patients encounter numerous respiratory problems and have poor clearance of their pulmonary secretions, all of which lead to repeated bouts of pneumonia and occasionally blood infections. If the cervical injury is below C5, then the patient can breathe independently and the long-term survival is improved. If the injury is at C6, the patient may have some shoulder (deltoid) function, which is controlled by the C5 root. Similarly, the root levels above the injury remain functional. With a C7 injury, the patient will have function of the biceps, and with the help of occupational therapy and attaching a spoon to a bracelet, the patient may even be able to lift the spoon to his/her mouth to feed and let gravity pull the arm down. All quadriplegic patients, however, will have a range of other problems that need continual attention. Because the legs and arms are immobile, they will form contractures that leave them contracted and very inflexible. This can limit any remaining function and needs physical therapy to preserve any residual flexibility. Because quadriplegics cannot move themselves and cannot feel pain, the skin and tissue underneath pressure points (buttocks, elbows, hips, back) can become eroded from the pressure, leading to exposed wounds. These wounds can be deep to the bone at times and need surgery to close. Untreated or undiagnosed wounds place the patient at risk for local infection and blood infection. As the function of the bladder and bowel are lost, quadriplegics will need to have indwelling catheters in the bladder. With time, these, too, lead to infections and surgeries become necessary to create secondary bladders. Other medical conditions affecting patients with paralysis include autonomic dysreflexia, chronic pain, and spasticity. See Table 15.

With injury to the thoracic spinal cord, breathing and arm function is preserved. However, in these paraplegic patients, the loss of movement in the trunk can severely affect the ability of the spine to stay upright while in a wheelchair. This is usually addressed by having a chest/belly strap that keeps one upright in the wheelchair, but the lower the level of injury, more abdominal muscle function is preserved, and accordingly less support is needed to stay upright. Because paraplegics cannot move their legs and hips and cannot feel pain, the skin and tissue underneath pressure points (buttocks, hips) can become eroded from the pressure, leading to exposed wounds. These wounds can be deep to the bone at times and need surgery to close. Untreated or undiagnosed wounds place the patient at risk for local infection and blood infection. As the function of the bladder and bowel is lost, quadriplegics and paraplegics will need to have indwelling catheters in the bladder, and, with time, these, too, lead to infections, and surgeries become necessary to create secondary bladders. See Table 16.

Table 15   Cervical spinal cord injury levels and loss of function

- C-3 vertebrae and above: Typically lose diaphragm function and require a ventilator to breathe.
- C-4: Have some use of biceps and shoulders, but weaker than C-5 and lower.
- C-5: May retain the use of shoulders and biceps, but not of the wrists or hands.
- C-6: Generally retain some wrist control, but no hand function.
- C-7 and T-1: Can usually straighten their arms but still may have dexterity problems with the hand and fingers. C-7 is the level for functional independence.

Spinal Cord Injury

Table 16   SCI medical problems

- **Urinary tract problems.** Nerves that run to the bladder can be affected by spinal cord injury resulting in the inability to control the release of urine, also known as urinary incontinence. Loss of bladder control can cause kidney infection, kidney or bladder stones, and increases your risk of urinary tract infections. Using a soft, thin tube you insert into your urethra and bladder to drain urine called a catheter, and drinking plenty of clear fluids several times a day can help.

- **Bowel management difficulties.** Voluntary control of the bowels may be lost or impaired after spinal cord injury. It can result in the inability to control your bowel movements, also known as fecal incontinence, or make it difficult for stool to move through your intestines. Bowel regulation can be aided by a high-fiber diet. Waste elimination can also be managed by available medications and other supplemental products.

- **Pressure sores.** Decubitus ulcers, bedsores, or pressure sores can be caused by sitting or lying in the same position for a long period of time. Spinal cord injury patients are especially susceptible to pressure sores because of reduced sensations, making the developing sore difficult to detect. The best way to prevent these sores is by changing positions frequently, with help, if necessary.

- **Deep vein thrombosis and pulmonary embolism.** Deep vein thrombosis occurs when decreased blood flow through the veins, usually due to sitting for long periods of time, cause blood clots to develop in a vein deep within a muscle. They can lead to a pulmonary embolism, a blocked pulmonary artery in the lungs. Spinal cord injury patients may need devices or medications to try and prevent clotting because large clots that block blood flow in this manner can be fatal.

- **Lung and breathing problems.** People with cervical and thoracic spinal cord injury may develop pneumonia, asthma, or other lung problems because it's more difficult to breathe and cough with weakened abdominal and chest muscles. These problems can be treated with medications and therapy. In some instances, people may need immunizations such as a yearly flu shot.

- **Autonomic dysreflexia.** Autonomic dysreflexia is a dangerous condition that can be caused by spinal cord injury above the middle of the chest where an irritation or pain below the level of the injury sends a signal that fails to reach the brain, producing a reflex action that can constrict blood vessels. A rise in blood pressure and a drop in heart rate results that can lead to stroke or seizure. Eliminating the cause of the irritation, which can be something as simple as a full bladder or tight clothes, or changing positions can help.

- **Spasticity.** Muscle spasms and jumping of the arms and legs can develop in some people with spinal cord injury. Unfortunately, this isn't an indication of recovery. The nerves in the lower spinal cord become more sensitive after injury and cause muscle contractions which manifest themselves in these exaggerated reflexes. The brain can no longer send signals to the lower nerves to regulate the contractions because of the spinal cord injury. If the spasms become severe, medical treatments may be necessary.

- **Weight control issues.** Muscle atrophy and weight loss are common after a spinal cord injury. Weight gain can also be caused by changes and lifestyle. This limits mobility, making it difficult for you to lift yourself, or be lifted from one place to another, and can also put you at risk for heart disease and other problems. Developing an exercise and diet plan with the assistance from a dietitian and rehabilitation therapist is a good idea.

(Continued)

Table 16 SCI medical problems *(continued)*

- **Sexual dysfunction.** Though many men, even those with little sensation in the genital area, suffering from spinal cord injury retain the ability to have erections, the erections may not last long enough or be firm enough for sexual activity. This can also affect fertility. Ninety percent of men with spinal cord injury lose the ability to ejaculate. However, this doesn't mean sexual activity, or fatherhood ceases to be an option for men with spinal cord injury. Solutions can be offered by doctors, urologists, and fertility specialists who specialize in spinal cord injury for better sexual functioning and fertility. Changes in sexuality and fertility can also affect women with spinal cord injury. Even though there is usually no change that inhibits sexual intercourse or pregnancy, some may lose the ability to produce vaginal lubrication or lose control of the vaginal muscles, and many experience changes in body image that affect sex drive. Additionally, it's important to consult a doctor before become pregnant as any pregnancy will be considered high risk.
- **Pain.** Pain inevitably results from accidents that damage to your spinal cord and other parts of your body. Areas of your body with little or no sensation can also feel pain. Overuse of muscles in an effort to compensate for impairment can also result in pain. For example, shoulder tendinitis from manually operating a wheelchair can develop over a long period of time. Any kind of pain will have a negative impact on daily living, and medications and modified activities can help manage this pain.
- **New injuries.** Spinal cord injury will increase your risk of injury to the areas of the body with impaired sensation. You may even experience a burn or cut without even realizing it. Inspect your body for any cuts or sores that need attention, and take steps to prevent new injuries.

45. What resources are available to me if I suffered a spinal cord injury?

Since the SCI suffered by Christopher Reeve, spinal cord injury has received more attention from both government and private agencies that offer support of those who are injured, as well as funding for research on SCI. For medical support, local doctors and hospitals will have counselors and managers to direct you to resources for prosthetics, physical therapy, occupational therapy, mental health counseling, as well as job placement.

Information can be found at your local libraries or more easily on the Web with a search for spinal cord injury. The National Institutes of Health and the Mayo Clinic have excellent Web sites with valuable information.

46. What research is ongoing regarding spinal cord injury?

Significant energy and resources are being directed toward SCI research. The research of treating a spinal cord injury is twofold. One form of research is being done to minimize the damage to the spinal cord at time of injury from secondary damage. This damage is from the inflammation at the injury site and from conditions that at the same time leave the patient with low blood pressure and low blood oxygenation levels. Minimizing the extent of acute injury is a high priority at trauma centers and hospitals that receive patients with SCI.

Scientists and doctors are trying to find ways to repair and regenerate the spinal cord so some function can be regained for patients with SCI.

The other major area of research is spinal cord regenerative medicine. Scientists and doctors are trying to find ways to repair and regenerate the spinal cord so some function can be regained for patients with SCI. The research includes the use of stem cells. With stem cells, the spinal cord neurons can be created in a laboratory dish and placed into the spinal cords of injured mice, leading to some recovery of function. Of course the application to humans is not here, but the results in animals are promising. Also, bioengineers are working on neural prostheses. These sophisticated devices are implanted under the skin and even in the brain to generate movement of the arms or a cursor on a computer screen.

PART SIX

Tumors of the Spine and Spinal Cord

What are the most common
tumors of the spinal cord?

What about metastatic disease to the spine?

How are spine and spinal cord tumors diagnosed?

More ...

47. What are the most common primary tumors of the spinal column?

Fortunately, the most common primary tumors to the spinal column are **benign**. Doctors use the term benign to indicate that a particular tumor is usually easy to control and that the patient is unlikely to die from this type of tumor. This is different from **malignant** tumors, which are more likely to spread, more difficult to control, and can be much more deadly.

The most common primary tumors of the spinal column are:

Osteoid osteomas—Osteoid osteomas are benign tumors that occur during the teenage years. Patients complain of severe pain that is usually well controlled with nonsteroidal anti-inflammatory drugs (NSAIDs) like ibuprofen. Diagnosis is made by bone scan and treatment includes NSAIDs, surgical excision, and a new treatment method using radio-frequency ablation. Evidence shows that with surgery or ablation the tumors rarely occurs.

Osteoblastomas—Osteoblastomas are essentially osteoid osteomas that are bigger than 2.0 cm in diameter. One difference is that they tend to have higher recurrence rates versus osteoid osteomas and because of their size usually require surgical resection.

Aneurysmal bone cysts—Aneurysmal bone cysts are rare benign tumors of the spine that tends to occur on the spinous processes and laminae of the spine. These lesions are treated with surgical resection if the spinal cord or spinal roots are compressed.

Benign

a tumor that is not cancerous or malignant. Benign lesions can still grow and cause damage to surrounding structures.

Malignant

a tumor that is cancerous or has the potential to spread to another part of the body. Tumors vary with respect to how malignant or aggressive they are.

Tumors of the Spine and Spinal Cord

Giant cell tumors—These tumors are benign by definition based on the behavior of their cells, but can be very aggressive and surgical resection is the main treatment. Their location tends to be in vertebral body (front of the spine).

Eosinophilic granuloma—An eosinophilic granuloma is a benign lesion that causes pain. On X-ray the finding can be very suggestive of this lesion when the vertebral body is flattened. These tumors can occurs as part of a syndrome of tumors that affect other parts of the body. Many of these tumors can be managed without surgery, or in certain cases with low-dose radiation.

Hemangioma—A hemangioma is a benign tumor that usually occurs in the vertebral body of the spine and is sometimes discovered while evaluating the spine for other diseases. If these lesions are leading to pain or other neurological symptoms, their treatment is surgical resection.

48. What are the most common tumors of the spinal cord?

The spinal cord is surrounded by dura and so when discussing tumors of the spinal cord they are categorized by being located in the substance of the spinal cord (called intradural and intramedullary) or by being located outside the substance of the spinal cord and still within the surrounding dura (called intradural and extramedullary). Intradural and extramedullary tumors are either nerve sheath tumors (schwannoma and neurofibroma) or meningiomas (Figure 21). Tumors within the dura and inside the substance of the spinal cord (intradural and extramedullary) are usually astrocytomas and ependymomas most commonly and occasionally hemangio-

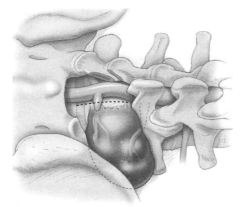

Figure 21   Extradural tumor of the spine.

blastomas, cavernomas, dermoids, epidermoids, lipomas, and others are even more uncommon.

Most spinal cord tumors are benign but because they are located in or by delicate structures most will need surgical resection. Usually patients have pain and after evaluation with imaging decisions are made about the need for observation, biopsy, and or resections. Malignant tumors of the spinal cord often require further treatment with radiation and/or chemotherapy.

49. What about metastatic disease to the spine?

Another category of spinal tumors is metastatic tumors. Tumor that arise outside of the spine can spread to other parts of the body. This spreading is called metastasis, and the spine because of the robust blood supply to the bone marrow within the spine make the spine a frequent location of metastasis.

Patients often complain of pain and many times the extent of surgical treatment for the spin metastasis depends

on potential longevity of patient. If the patient has limited lifespan this should be considered when deciding
on the surgical plan. However, many spine metastases
need surgical resection or intervention to prevent collapse of spine or alleviation of compression. Radiation
therapy can be effective as well.

50. How are spine and spinal cord tumors diagnosed?

Tumors of the spine and spinal cord are relatively uncommon. The most common initial symptom that patients with a spinal tumor have is pain. Because back
pain is very common, it is also not a specific symptom
of any one disease or medical condition. Spinal tumors
can be either primary (originating in the spine) or secondary (metastases of cancer that originated elsewhere
in the body). Therefore, the challenge is to determine
how to evaluate back pain with the goal of specifically
excluding a tumor as the cause of the pain. Luckily,
most back pain is not due to a tumor. However, if a
cancer were discovered after a long period of conservative management of back pain, most patients would
feel that their problem should have been investigated
more thoroughly in the beginning. Magnetic resonance
imaging (MRI) is the imaging study of choice to evaluate spinal tumors.

51. What is the best treatment for a spine tumor?

The best treatment for a spine tumor depends on the
type of tumor. In general, surgery is the most effective
treatment for most benign spinal column tumors and all
intradural neoplasms. Long-term control or cure can
be achieved with total removal of the extramedullary

tumors and the majority of intramedullary neoplasms. Thus, early diagnosis and aggressive initial surgery provide the best opportunity for long, progression-free survival. Subsequent surgery is generally more difficult due to scarring.

For malignant or metastatic tumors of the spine, a combination of surgery, radiation therapy (or radiosurgery), and chemotherapy are usually recommended. Many metastatic lesions that were once treated with radiation alone are amenable to surgery. In recent years, surgery plus radiation has been shown to be more effective than radiation alone. Furthermore, surgery may correct a deformity caused by the tumor and remove pressure on the spinal cord, allowing a person to continue to walk and maintain function of bladder and bowel.

In recent years, surgery plus radiation has been shown to be more effective than radiation alone.

52. What is spinal radiosurgery?

Radiosurgery is a term used to refer to a class of radiation techniques that are spatially very precise and enables radiation to be delivered to delicate areas of the body. This approach makes it possible to administer aggressive doses of radiation without damaging adjacent normal tissue. To achieve the above objectives, radiosurgery is delivered in a small number of treatments (usually 1 or 2). This type of radiotherapy has gained popularity for treating certain spine tumors, due to their proximity to the spinal cord. Both benign (noncancerous) and malignant (cancerous or capable of spreading to other sites in the body) spinal tumors can be treated with spinal radiosurgery.

53. What is a spondylectomy?

A **spondylectomy** is a surgical procedure in which the surgeon removes a vertebra. Since the vertebra encircles

Spondylectomy

the complete removal of a spinal vertebra through a surgical procedure. It is commonly performed for removal of a tumor. Following spondylectomy, the spine is usually stabilized with hardware.

85

the spinal cord, the vertebra must be removed in two pieces, using advanced surgical techniques. A spondylectomy is recommended for certain types of spine tumors that are confined to the vertebra. This technique is highly specialized but often provides patients with the optimal chance for cure of certain types of spine tumors.

PART SEVEN

Scoliosis

What is idiopathic scoliosis?

How is scoliosis diagnosed?

What if scoliosis is left untreated?

More . . .

54. What is idiopathic scoliosis?

The normal and healthy spine has curves. When the curve is side-to-side while looking at the spine from front to back it is considered abnormal and called scoliosis (Figure 22). By itself scoliosis doesn't denote a disease but is more a descriptive term. When the curve becomes excessive (as measure by the clinician on X-rays; see Figure 23) there is risk of worsening curvature.

The causes of scoliosis are various and the treatments depend on the cause as well as degree of scoliosis. Idiopathic scoliosis is the most common type of scoliosis in

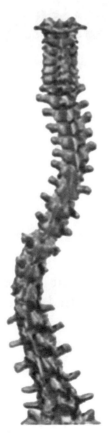

Figure 22   Thoracic scoliosis.

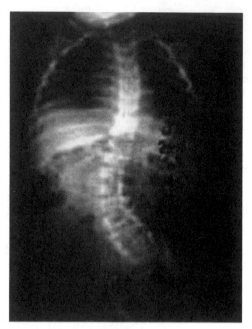

Figure 23 X-ray of thoracic and lumbar scoliosis.

America and Canada with diagnosis usually occurring during adolescence and most commonly in girls. The treatment can be bracing for less severe scoliosis and surgery when the curve has certain measurements excluding if from brace treatment.

55. What is degenerative scoliosis?

Degenerative scoliosis occurs in adults and is the result of cumulative wear and tear on the spine. This degeneration of the spine can lead to scoliosis and is exacerbated by the compounding effects of osteoporosis and prior spine surgery. This type of scoliosis usually occurs after the age of 40.

Patients have back and leg pain with with weakness, numbness, or tingling. The complaints vary between patients and need to be separated from other causes of back and leg pain. The usual treatment is conservative with exercise, weight loss, pain medicines and physical therapy.

For those patients in whom the pain can't be controlled or neurological signs (such as leg pain, weakness, or numbness) are becoming worse, surgery for decompression or nerver roots and correction of the scoliosis deformity can be very helpful. Depending on the degree of problems surgical options range from decompression with laminectomy and/or deformity correction with spinal instrumentation.

56. How is scoliosis diagnosed?

Most cases are scoliosis are diagnosed during adolescence when the abnormal spine curve becomes more noticeable. Regardless of the cause of scoliosis, the diagnosis and evaluation is aided by a complete history from the patient and imaging of the spine.

Your doctor may ask about:

- Is there any family history of scoliosis?
- When was the first time the abnormal spine curve was noticed?
- Do you have pain or weakness?
- Have you had any changes in urination or defecation?
- Have you had any previous surgery?

The complete history is aided by a complete physical exam performed by the clinician. Ultimately, a variety of imaging may be ordered to further define any scoliosis and can include plain X-rays (which are usually standing and bending, as well as from the front and side). A CT scan may be ordered as well. Further an MRI can provide necessary information about the spinal cord and nerve roots. Taken together, the history, physical exam and medical imaging provides the information from which your clinician can diagnose and make a treatment plan for scoliosis.

57. How is scoliosis classified?

There are many types of scoliosis, each with its own classification system. The most common classification schemes are for adolescent idiopathic scoliosis (AIS). The classification schemes take into account the angle of the curve (also known as the Cobb angle), the coronal balance (whether your shoulders are centered over your hips), and the sagittal balance (whether your neck is centered over your tailbone). The classification schemes are rather detailed, but your physician will mostly be concerned with progression over time, where your body has compensated well for a particular curve, and the degree of the curve. All these factors lead in the decision making with respect to conservative therapy (bracing and physical therapy) or surgery.

The treatment of scoliosis is highly varied and can include the following: physical therapy, activity modification, bracing, pain medications, and surgery.

58. How is scoliosis treated?

The treatment of scoliosis is highly varied and can include the following: physical therapy, activity modification, bracing, pain medications, and surgery. The treatment plan, which may include surgery, is dependent on many variables including the type of scoliosis, the age of the patient, and the degree of scoliosis. Treatment includes:

Monitoring: Most patients will have their scoliosis monitored with serial imaging take every 4 to 12 months. The clinician will decide the frequency and type of imaging with which to monitor the patient.

Physical Therapy: Physical therapy is very helpful in most types of scoliosis and can relieve pain and help build the supporting musculature. A rehabilitation program can also help with increasing mobility and strength.

Bracing: The use of bracing is a very important option in the treatment of scoliosis. When scoliosis is of a limited degree and not severe enough for surgery, bracing can help prevent the progression of scoliosis. The brace needs to be worn for a minimum number of hours.

Surgery: Surgery is a treatment option for hard to control pain, disfigurement, worsening curve, and/or problems with breathing. Even when surgery is the treatment plan, physical therapy, exercise, and bracing is often used before and after surgery.

59. What if scoliosis is left untreated?

Once scoliosis is diagnosed, concern about whether the curves will continue to grow bigger may arise. There is no absolute way to tell, but this much is known:

- Curves in the thoracic spine are more likely to progress than lumbar curves.
- The likelihood of progression is linked to the size of the curve. Larger curves are more likely to get bigger.
- If the curves start at a young age or before a girl begins her period, they are more likely to progress.
- Even though it is recommended for severe cases, a patient may choose not to have surgery because of

the risks. There are risks of leaving large curves untreated such as:

Increased back pain—Patients with untreated large curves can suffer from daily back pain.

Reduced respiratory function—Large curves lead to deformities that can lower the space for the body's vital organs, such as the lungs and heart. The reduction in space can compromise the ability to breathe and for the heart to function properly. In curves of 100 degrees or more, the affects can be life threatening.

PART EIGHT

Pediatric Spine Disorders

What is a tethered cord?

What is spina bifida, and
what is a neural tube defect?

At what age do pediatric spine disorders present?

More ...

60. What is a tethered cord?

Tethered spinal cord syndrome is a neurological disorder caused by stretching of the spinal cord as a child grows. The spinal cord is attached to the tail bone region to limit the movement of the spinal cord within the spinal column. Sometimes the connection to this region doesn't loosen sufficiently as the spinal canal expands and leaves a constant stretch on the spinal cord, hence it is called a tethered spinal cord. The disorder is progressive as the child grows. Symptoms may include lesions, hairy patches, dimples, or fatty tumors on the lower back, foot and spinal deformities, weakness or paralysis in the legs, low back pain, and incontinence. In older children scoliosis may develop. Tethered spinal cord syndrome may go undiagnosed until late childhood or adulthood, when sensory and motor problems and loss of bowel and bladder control emerge. This delayed presentation of symptoms is related to the degree of strain placed on the spinal cord over time. Tethering may also develop after spinal cord injury and scar tissue can block the flow of fluids around the spinal cord.

61. What is spina bifida, and what is a neural tube defect?

A neural tube defect is a disorder involving the failure of a fetus's neural tube to close during pregnancy. The neural tube is what later develops into the brain, spinal cord, and their protective coverings. Neural tube defects occur in the first month of pregnancy. Spina bifida is a neural tube defect occurring in the spine. A baby born with spina bifida may have an open lesion on his/her spine where significant damage to the nerves and spinal cord has occurred, and often the spinal cord and nerves are exposed. Although the spinal opening can be surgically repaired shortly after birth, the nerve damage may be permanent, resulting in varying degrees of paralysis of the lower limbs. In the mildest forms, patients may not have any noticeable neurologic injury. However, more commonly, patients have some degree of neurologic injury and often complete paralysis. Even when there is no lesion present, there may be improperly formed or missing vertebrae and accompanying nerve damage. In addition to physical and mobility difficulties, most individuals have some form of learning disability. The three most common types of spina bifida are myelomeningocele, meningocele, and spina bifida occulta. Myelomeningocele, the severest form, is when the spinal cord and its protective covering (the meninges) protrude from an opening in the spine. Meningocele occurs when the spinal cord develops normally but the meninges protrude from a spinal opening. Spina bifida occulta is the mildest and most common form; in this form, one or more vertebrae are malformed and covered by a layer of skin, but the spinal cord and nerve roots aren't exposed. There is often a tuft of hair, a skin dimple, or a suspicious mole overlying the spine at that area. Spina bifida may also cause bowel and bladder complications, and many children with spina bifida develop a condition called hydrocephalus (excessive accumulation of cerebrospinal fluid in the brain).

Unfortunately, there is no cure for spina bifida because the nerve tissue cannot be replaced or repaired. Treatment for the variety of effects of spina bifida may include surgery, medication, and physiotherapy. Many individuals with spina bifida will need assistive devices such as braces, crutches, or wheelchairs. Ongoing therapy, medical care, and/or surgical treatments may be necessary to prevent and manage complications throughout the individual's life. Surgery to close the newborn's spinal opening is generally performed by a neurosurgeon within 24 hours after birth to minimize the risk of infection and to preserve existing function in the spinal cord.

62. How are pediatric spine disorders diagnosed?

Pediatric spine disorders are difficult to diagnose. A prenatal ultrasound may alert an obstetrician or pediatrician to certain spinal disorders such as spina bifida. On a newborn, physical exam findings, such as an unusual tuft of hair, a deep skin dimple, or an abnormal mole overlying the spine may alert the pediatrician to a possible underlying spine disorder. As babies get older, difficulty crawling, standing, or walking or recurrent urinary infections may also be a sign of a spine disorder. Older children are diagnosed with spine disorders through scoliosis screening, obvious physical deformity, or through a routine neurologic examination as part of a checkup. Older children are also able to describe symptoms, including pain, which may alert a family member of a problem.

Most diagnoses are made by clinical criteria. However, MRI is also extremely valuable in diagnosing many severe spinal disorders in children.

63. At what age do pediatric spine disorders present?

Pediatric spine disorders present anywhere from birth through adulthood. Neural tube defects and spina bifida are diagnosed during pregnancy or at time of birth. Tethered spinal cord is usually diagnosed before age 5, but mild forms might not become symptomatic until early adulthood. Scoliosis, which makes up the majority of pediatric spine disorders, is usually diagnosed in the early teen years, during a time of rapid spine growth. Spine tumors present at any age in childhood, but rarely before 1 year of age.

64. How are pediatric spine disorders treated?

Fortunately, many pediatric spine disorders are mild and do not require surgery for treatment. The severity of the disorder will dictate the optimal treatment. After the diagnosis is made, your physician will determine the severity of symptoms and the underlying problem through a combination of physical examination, imaging studies, and physiologic tests of muscle and bladder function (**urodynamics**). Mild forms are generally treated with conservative therapy including observation, physical therapy, and bracing. Occasionally activity limitations may need to be imposed. If symptoms do not resolve, or if progression of disease is noted, surgery may be required. Surgery on the spine is generally safe with the aid of advanced technology such as an operating microscope, neuromonitoring, and fluoroscopy. Surgery is generally reserved for the most severe disorders, but if performed properly, it can treat disorders with a high degree of success.

Urodynamics

a series of tests used to evaluate the neurological function of the urinary system. Severe injury to the low back may cause urinary problems and urodynamics may help assess the degree of damage.

65. What are urodynamics?

Urodynamics are a set of tests used to assess the function of the lower urinary tract, namely the bladder and urethra. They use physical measurements such as urine pressure and flow rate as well as clinical assessment by a physician.

The assessment begins with a medical history and examination, which may, for example, reveal abnormalities within the lower abdomen or pelvis that are contributing to the lower urinary tract symptoms.

The patient (or his/her parent) is then given a urination (voiding) diary to be kept for 3 days to document fluid intake and output, including episodes of incontinence. This provides information about bladder capacity, the frequency of passage of urine, and episodes of incontinence and getting up at night to urinate. The diary can also outline other problems such as excessive fluid intake. Then formal urodynamics studies are done. Urodynamics can help determine if urinary abnormalities are due to primary neurologic injury, such as a tethered spinal cord. Often, these are the first signs, and they help alert your physician to potential problems before they happen.

66. What are some of the congenital disorders of the spine?

Congenital disorders of the spine are disorders that are due to a development defect during the 4th to 6th week of gestation (pregnancy). Congenital kyphosis is a failure of proper spinal column formation. Congenital scoliosis, an abnormally curved spine, is the most common congenital spinal disorder.

PART NINE

Diagnostic Studies

What is the typical history
for a patient with spine disease?

What is a CT scan?

What is a myelogram?

More ...

67. What is the typical history for a patient with spine disease?

The symptoms of a patient who presents with spine disease depend upon the location and severity of the disease. Spine disease is most common in the neck and low back but can occur anywhere in the spine from the base of the skull to the tailbone. The most common symptoms are neck pain, low back pain, shooting arm or leg pain, reduced range of motion in the neck or back, abnormal posture, weakness in the arms or legs, numbness in the arms or legs, difficulty walking or using the legs, and difficulty writing or using the hands.

Most people suffer neck or back pain at some point in their life. However, if the pain is extreme, or particularly if it is associated with neurologic injury (i.e., numbness or weakness in an arm or leg), spine disease may be present. Often mild symptoms subside on their own, with rest, or with conservative therapy (i.e., physical therapy). However, if symptoms persist or get worse, more invasive treatments such as injections or surgery may be necessary to treat the pain and prevent further damage.

Most people suffer neck or back pain at some point in their life.

68. What are physical exam findings in patients with spine disease?

In patients with spine disease the physical exam can provide important information to the what type of spine disease is responsible as well as the timing and urgency in which the treatment should be implemented.

The clinician will ask you about:

- Do you have pain?
- Where does the pain start and finish?

Diagnostic Studies

- What makes the pain better of worse?
- Is the pain associated with twisting or bending?
- Do you have muscle spasms and where?

Then the spine will be examined for the following:

- Ability to bend and rotate your neck.
- Ability to bend and rotate your lower back.
- Checked for areas of tenderness.

Also, the spinal cord and spinal nerve root function will be examined:

- Evaluating for numbness on the arms, legs, and trunk.
- Testing for reflexes.
- Testing for various types of sensation.

69. What are X-rays?

An X-ray (see Figure 24) is an imaging test that uses a radioactive beam to take pictures of bone. The beam is projected through your body onto a special film, just like a camera.

An X-ray is good at showing bone. An X-ray is helpful if your doctor suspects a fracture of the spine, an infection, or a tumor. Doctors have used X-rays for over 100 years to check bone alignment and to see whether certain shadows appear to be out of alignment. This can give them clues about the health of soft tissues around the spine. If your doctor thinks your problem may be from degeneration of the spine, X-rays can be used to see if the space between your vertebrae is decreased, if there are bone spurs, or if there is an overgrowth of the joints.

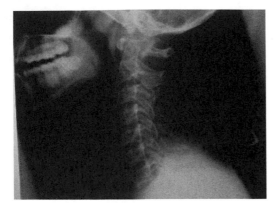

Figure 24   X-ray of the cervical spine.

Having an X-ray is much like having your photograph taken. It is a quick and painless procedure. You will be asked to lie very still on a table or stand very still and hold certain positions while pictures are taken of your spine. Sometimes X-rays are taken while you are in different positions. For example, an X-ray may be taken while you bend forward (flexion), and another while you straighten your spine (extension). This is called a flexion-extension view of the spine. These X-rays are compared to see if there is extra movement between the vertebrae, a condition called segmental instability.

X-rays are not good at showing the soft tissues—nerves, discs, and ligaments. Today, many tests can show the soft tissues much clearer, so doctors do not always have to rely on X-rays. However, X-rays provide a good starting point in evaluating the spine.

X-rays use radiation, which in large doses can increase the risks of cancer. The vast majority of patients who get

X-rays will never get enough radiation to worry about cancer. Only patients who must have large numbers—hundreds—of X-rays over many years need to worry about this risk. Children and young adults who plan to have children should be protected from radiation exposure to the testicles and ovaries. The radiation can damage the sperm and eggs. It is simple to protect these areas by shielding them with a lead apron or lead blanket.

Carrie's comments:

My doctors were great because they were able to walk me through all the imaging and explain exactly what was going on. They showed me on a conventional X-ray my L5, and it was striking how out of place it was from the rest of my spine. I remember being really shocked, and still am, that something so drastic was happening in my body. I guess I sort of knew all along that something was amiss with all the symptoms, but seeing the imaging made it all of a sudden so real.

70. What is a CT scan?

The CT or CAT scan (Figure 25) is an X-ray test that shows bones and soft tissues. The abbreviation CAT stands for computer-assisted tomography. X-rays are taken and then interpreted by a powerful computer that makes them appear as slices through the body. Special computer software can combine these images into a three-dimensional view of the bones.

The slices produced by a CT scan allow each section of the spine to be examined separately. The images show details of spine bones in great detail. A CT scan can show if bone spurs are pushing against spinal nerve roots. It is often used when looking at fractures or damaged bones due to infection or cancer. Some doctors

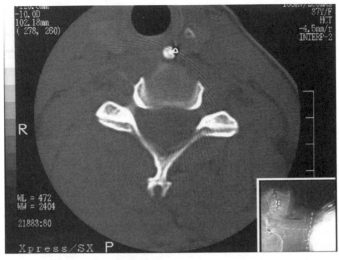

Figure 25   CT scan of cervical spine.

have recently begun using CT scan technology on a limited basis to test for osteoporosis in the spine.

When undergoing the test, you will be asked to lie on a table that slides into a scanner. This is similar to having an MRI test. The scanner used for CT scans is essentially an X-ray tube that rotates in a circle. You will need to lie very still for short periods while the scanner takes many pictures. The procedure takes 30–60 minutes.

The limitations of CT are that it does not show muscles or ligaments clearly. To make the nerves and soft tissues easier to see, this test is often combined with a **myelogram**. With the myelogram, dye is injected into the spinal sac to outline the nerves and spinal sac so they show up clearly on the CT scan. A CT scan without dye is not as good at showing the discs and the nerves of the spine. The CT scan was developed before magnetic resonance imaging (MRI). The pictures of soft tissues are not as clear as they are with an MRI. The MRI is a better test to show problems within the disc, particular-

Myelogram

a test in which dye is injected into the spinal sac around the spinal cord and various X-rays are taken. The test is often used to evaluate for spinal compression in patients who cannot undergo MRI.

109

ly a recurring disc herniation. It is also helpful for showing the health of a disc following surgery.

The risks of CT are the same as X-rays. In large doses, radiation from the CT scan OKcan increase the risk of cancer. The vast majority of patients who have a CT scan will never get enough radiation to worry about cancer. Only patients who must have large numbers—hundreds—of X-rays or CT scans over many years need to be concerned. Children and young adults who plan to have children should be protected from radiation exposure to the testicles and ovaries. Otherwise the radiation may damage the sperm and eggs. It is simple to protect these areas by shielding them with a lead apron or lead blanket.

71. What is an MRI?

Magnetic resonance imaging (MRI) is one typing of imaging for the spine that is particularly useful evaluating soft tissue (such as discs and ligaments) and the spinal cord and roots. It uses magnetic wave technology to generate images without using radiation. It is frequently used to evaluate a wide variety of spine disease. (see Figure 26).

The MRI can show detailed anatomy of the general spine with particularly useful information about the shape and condition of the vertebral discs as well has any wear and tear of the ligaments.

The MRI is performed with the patient lying down and passing though a large round tunnel and can often be noisy. The test can last from 15 to 45 minutes depending on the type of MRI and for patients that have anxiety, often some mild medication can be given.

Patients with metal implants (not titanium used in spinal instrumentation) can lead to serious problems

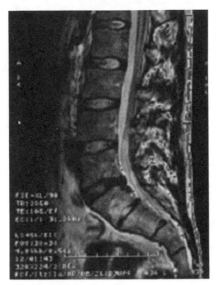

Figure 26   MRI of lumbar spine.

and need to discuss in detail with the doctor or technician if they have metal clips in their bodies (from prior surgery) or if they have a pacemaker. Most current implants for patients are MRI compatible.

72. What is a myelogram?

A myelogram is another test that can be used to evaluate the spine and spinal cord. Unlike an MRI, it has an invasive component. A dye is placed into the spinal fluid by injection and an X-ray is taken. In some cases a CT scan of the spine can be taken to provide more detail. The dye allows for the evaluation of spinal cord root shape and any compression that may be present. Because the myelogram requires a spinal tap, there are more risks associated with it than most other tests.

This test is especially usefull in patients who cannot receive an MRI (metal implants that are incompatible) or for patients in which and MRI fails to provide useful information.

Because the myelogram requires a spinal tap, there are more risks associated with it than most other tests.

111

73. What is a discogram?

A **discogram** (Figure 27) is a test that allows better evaluation of disc shape and whether pain is potentially originating from a particular disc. During a discogram, dye is injected into the intervertebral discs and visualize using X-ray technology.

Once the dye is injected into the disc the clinician will ask you about any pain that you are having and whether this pain is similar to the back and/or leg pain you usually have. Based on the reproduction of pain and the shape of the disc on discogram your clinician can gain more information about the source of your pain.

This test is invasive and requires injection into the intervertebral risks. As such there are small risks of infection and complications. The test usually takes 30–60 minutes. During the test you may receive medicine to relieve anxiety and help you relax during the procedure.

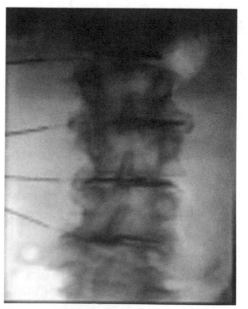

Figure 27   **Discogram of lumbar spine.**

74. What is a bone scan?

A bone scan is a test that reveals areas of the spine that may have a altered metabolism, which is seen in cancer, bone fractures, and infection. The test involves injecting a radioactive chemical (at doses that are safe) into the bloodstream, which goes to areas of increased metabolism in the bone. Several hours later a picture is taken with a special camera that shows these "hot" spots.

A bone scan is very useful when the cause of your spine disease is unclear and when supporting evidence is sought by your clinician for a diagnosis he may be suspecting. The risks are related to potential dye allergy and are very low.

Diagnostic Studies

PART TEN

Nonsurgical Treatment

What is spinal physical therapy?

What medications or supplements may help?

What is a facet injection or nerve block?

More …

75. What is spinal physical therapy?

Physical therapy is one of the non-surgical treatments that can help patient with spine disease. This can be used in place of surgery for some conditions and along with surgery for many conditions. Physical therapy is exercise and lifestyle changes that help with creating or maintaining a healthy spine. The muscles that support your spine are strengthened to take some of the pressure off the spine and posture is improved to help take pressure off the spine as well.

A physical therapist (PT) will help train and educate you and this can occur in the hospital as well as at out-patient facilities. After evaluating you your PT may recommend one or more of the following interventions:

- Ways to improve your posture
- *Help define how much work and how much rest is necessary*
- Ice treatment
- Heat treatment
- Electrical or ultrasound treatment
- Massage
- Traction (using devices and positional techniques to stretch your spine and temporarily relieve some compression of spinal joints and nerves)
- Strength training to help provide better support to the spine
- *Body mechanics*—Thinking about the way you use your body to perform tasks during the day that will prevent strain on your spine:

  - Plan and prepare for the lift.
  - Make sure you have good footing.
  - Straddle your feet with a wide base of support.
  - Keep the load close.

- Keep the spine stable and aligned.
- Avoid twisting by pivoting with your feet.
- Bend at the knees and instead of your waist
- Use your thighs and legs to lift not your back

- *Ergonomics*—Learning to work with proper positioning and having the work environment designed with ergonomics in mind.

Richard's comments:

I went through physical therapy initially as part of my preoperative treatment for pain, and also as part of surgical rehabilitation. These sessions involved a lot of stretching, as expected, but also involved a lot of muscle-building exercises that helped strengthen my back muscles. My pain did go away for a bit after each therapy session (replaced by a pleasant soreness), but never fully subsided, and soon just kept getting worse. After surgery, therapy really helped speed up my recovery. I never would have gotten back to work so quickly without it. It ended up being quite a workout, similar to yoga, except more directed movements. I found some muscles I didn't even know I had!

76. What is conservative treatment?

Conservative treatment is essentially all the methods that are available to help patients with spine disease that don't involve surgery or procedures. This includes, but is not limited to pain management, physical therapy, rest, bracing, traction, as well as less conventional methods of acupressure, acupuncture and biofeedback. In general conservative management doesn't place the patient at any risk and has the potential to provide pain relief and improve disability. Often once conservative management fails, surgery is considered the next option. One caveat is that many types of spine disease should be treated with surgery first and conservative management is not indicated.

Richard's comments:

My doctors advised me that they would first try conservative treatment. They put me through a physical therapy regimen and medicated me with the pain to see if there was any chance I would get enough relief to avoid surgery. Though this was not the case, I certainly appreciate the efforts they took to keep me from going under the knife. While my outcome was ultimately a good one, at the time I was also very keen on avoiding an operation at all costs, and was willing to try anything.

77. What medications or supplements may help?

Mild pain medications can reduce inflammation and pain when taken properly. Pain medications cannot stop the effects of aging and wear and tear on the spine, but they can help control pain. If you are pregnant, you should not take any medication unless you have discussed it with your obstetrician.

General Tips

- Medications should be used wisely. Take them exactly as prescribed by your doctor and report any side effects.
- Some pain medications are highly addictive.
- Pain medication is less effective for controlling chronic pain if used over a long period.
- Medication will not cure pain of degenerative origin.

Medications prescribed for back pain include:

- *Aspirin*—Aspirin compounds are over-the-counter medications that can help relieve minor pain and backache. The main potential side effect with aspirin is the development of stomach problems—particularly ulcers with or without bleeding.

- *NSAIDs*—Nonsteroidal anti-inflammatory drugs (NSAIDs) include over-the-counter pain relievers such as ibuprofen and naproxen. These medications were once only available by prescription. NSAIDs are very effective in relieving the pain associated with muscle strain and inflammation. Be aware that NSAIDs can decrease renal function if you are an older patient. Excessive use can lead to kidney problems.

- *COX-2 inhibitors*—A new class of NSAIDs is gaining wide acceptance in its ability to reduce inflammation. Commonly called COX-2 inhibitors, these newer NSAIDS work by selectively blocking the formation of pain-causing inflammatory chemicals. COX-2 inhibitors appear to be easier on the stomach, mainly because they don't interrupt stomach enzymes like traditional NSAIDs. Celecoxib (Celebrex) and rofecoxib (Vioxx) are two commonly prescribed COX-2 inhibitors. Recent concern over side effects related to the heart has arisen; you should discuss this in detail with your physician before taking these medications.

- *Nonnarcotic prescription pain medications*—Nonnarcotic analgesics (pain relievers) are ideal in the treatment of mild to moderate chronic pain. Acetaminophen and aspirin are the most widely used over-the-counter analgesics. Medications that are analgesics and require a prescription from the doctor include NSAIDs, such as carprofen, fenoprofen, ketoprofen, and sulindac. To reduce side effects, do not lie down for 15–30 minutes after taking the medication, avoid direct sunlight, and wear protective clothing and sun block. Avoid using these medications if you have recurrent ulcers or liver problems.

- *Narcotic pain medications*—If you experience severe pain, your doctor might prescribe a narcotic pain medication such as codeine or morphine. Narcotics relieve pain by acting as a numbing anesthetic to the central nervous system. The strength and length of pain relief differs for each drug.

    Narcotics can have side effects such as nausea, vomiting, constipation, and sedation (drowsiness). These side effects are predictable and can often be prevented. Common preventive measures include not taking sleeping aids or antidepressants along with narcotics, avoiding alcohol, increasing fluid intake, eating a high-fiber diet, and using a fiber laxative or stool softener to treat constipation. Remember that narcotics can be addictive if used excessively or improperly.

- *Muscle relaxants*—If you are having muscle spasms, muscle relaxants may help relieve pain. However, they have only been shown to be marginally effective. Muscle relaxants also have a significant risk of drowsiness and depression. Long-term use is not suggested; only 3–4 days is typically recommended.

- *Antidepressants*—Back pain is a common symptom of depression and could be an indicator of its presence. Similarly, back pain can lead to emotional distress and depression. It seems that the same chemical reactions in the nerve cells that trigger depression also control the pain pathways in the brain. Antidepressants can relieve emotional stress associated with back pain. Some antidepressant medications seem to reduce pain—probably because they affect this chemical reaction in the nerve cells.

    Some types of antidepressants make good sleeping medications. If you are having trouble sleeping due to your back pain, your doctor may prescribe an antidepressant to help you get back to a normal sleep routine. Antidepressants can have side effects such as drowsiness, loss of appetite, constipation, dry mouth, and fatigue.

- *Nutritional supplements*—Nutritional supplements may help the body in the healing process following a spine injury. Proper diet and exercise increase their effectiveness. Recently, joint supplements such as glucosamine and chondroitin have come on the market. They may be beneficial for some types of spinal joint disorders.

Richard's comments:

By the time I decided to see a doctor about my back pain, I had already worked my way though all the over-the-counter pain medications (acetaminophen, ibuprofen, etc.). My doctor put me on some prescription painkillers that worked for awhile, but the pain came back. After a few more weeks of pain, I opted for the surgery. In the meantime, my doctor put me on some more powerful narcotic drugs that worked wonders for a short period of time, but left me feeling a little incapacitated at times.

78. What is a brace?

A brace is something you wear on the outside of your body that restricts motion of the spine to varying degrees. Essentially it holds the spine still, and prevents worsening of a fracture, alleviates pain associated with movement, and in some cases allows fractures to heal.

In the neck various braces can be used as prescribed by your clinican:

- *Soft collar* (Figure 28)—This is actually not a brace and worn for comfort, but doesn't provide any real support of the cervical spine. It can be used as a transition to wearing no collar or brace at all.

Nonsurgical Treatment

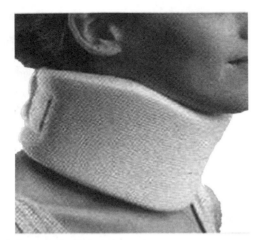

Figure 28   Soft cervical collar.

- *Philadelphia collar* (Figure 29)—This is a rigid brace that wraps around your neck and is held in place with Velcro straps, preventing you from bending your neck. This brace will hold the cervical spine still and is commonly used for fractures, post-surgery, and cervical strain. A similar type is the Miami cervical brace (Figure 30).
- *Sterno-occipital mandibular immobilization device (SOMI)*—A SOMI (Figures 31 and 32) is a brace

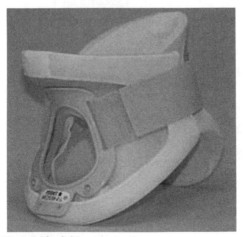

Figure 29   Philadelphia rigid cervical collar.

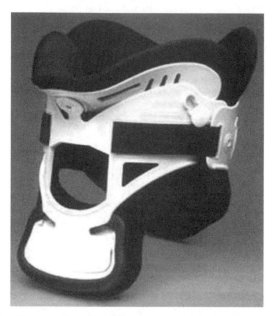

Figure 30   Miami rigid cervical collar.

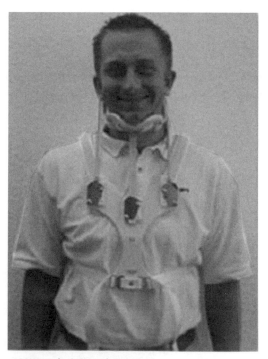

Figure 31   SOMI cervical thoracic brace.

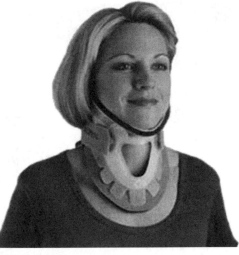

Figure 32   SOMI cervical brace.

not only wraps around your neck, but also is attached to your chest. This prevents the neck from bending or twisting relative to the shoulders. This brace provides great support for the cervical spine and is used in special clinical cases.

- *Halo* (Figure 33)—The halo is a rigid cervical brace that provides excellent support for the cervical spine by attaching the head to the shoulders with the use of a ring and rods. This is the most rigid of the cervical braces. A ring is secured around the top of your head with pins and the ring is connected to a vest with rods. This is worn around the clock and the pins used to fix the halo ring to the head need to be routinely cleaned with antiseptic.

For the thoracic and lumbar spine several braces exist as well:

Corsets (Figure 34). Corsets provide support for the back and limit movement. These braces are similar to

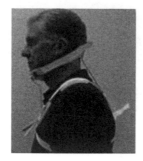
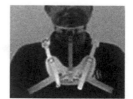
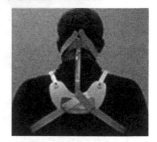

Figure 33   Rigid cervical brace.

the soft collar for the cervical spine in that they don't provide enough rigidity to prevent movement in the spine. But they do limit some movement so they have application for limiting back pain or as a transition brace when moving out of a rigid brace.

Rigid braces (Figure 35) are used for instability and fractures of the thoracic and lumbar spine. These rigid

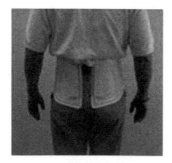
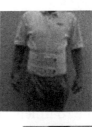
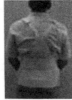

Figure 34   Rigid lumbar brace (corset).

Nonsurgical Treatment

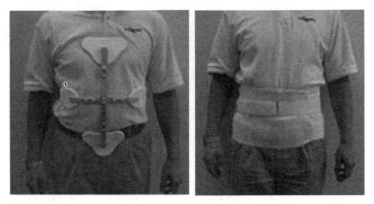

Figure 35   CASH (left) and molded (right) rigid lumbar braces.

corsets extend from across the chest and down to the pelvis. Many patients state that these braces look like turtle shells, which hold the trunk and lower back rigidly. These are fitted to individual patients and have to be worn around the clock. X-rays are usually taken with the brace on an patient standing to make sure that the fractured or post-surgical spine is not getting worse. If it isn't then the brace is used for at least 6 weeks and sometimes more.

79. What is an epidural steroid injection?

Spinal injections are procedures done to the spine that can treat pain for a limited period of time. Since the risks of this procedure are very low, they are often used by patients who are not yet candidates for surgery. Also, if a spinal injection relieves your pain, it provides more evidence toward which part of the spine is the source of pain and likely target for surgical intervention.

Epidural spinal injections essentially place numbing medicine over the spinal cord and roots creating pain relief, sometimes up to weeks. They are called epidural, because the numbing medicine and anti-inflammatory medicine is place outside of the dura (covering of the spinal cord and roots) and directly over the spinal root and spinal cord.

There are several techniques by which epidural injections can be performed:

- *Caudal block*—Placing the numbing medicine over the lumbosacral region.
- *Translumbar*—Injecting between two vertebral bodies and into the epidural space
- *Transforaminal*—Injecting through the holes from which the spinal nerve roots exit. This is a very selective placement of medicine and often is used for diagnostic purposes.

80. What is a facet injection or nerve block?

Facet joints are the joints that connect the vertebral levels by connecting laminae to adjoining levels. Like other joint in the body, facet joint can become inflamed and irritated contributing to back pain. With a facet injection a needle is inserted into your facet from the back and numbing medicine is injected. Relief of pain is a strong suggestive that the facet is contributing to the pain and provide useful information to the surgeon about which operation has the best chance of success.

Risks of infection are associated with this procedure because the joint is entered, however the risks are very low. This test is especially useful if the information provided by other non-invasive tests is inconclusive.

81. What is traction?

Spinal traction uses manually or mechanically created forces to stretch and mobilize the spine in an attempt to treat nerve root compression and spine pain. Traction may alleviate back pain by stretching tight spinal muscles that result from spasm and widen intervertebral foramen to relieve nerve root impingement.

Each patient is unique and what works well for one patient may not be appropriate for another. Therefore, each prospective patient is carefully evaluated prior to treatment. This assessment enables the therapist to make decisions about the type of traction to be utilized, the force/weight of distraction, and the duration of treatment.

The goal of traction is to reduce pain to assist the patient to become more functional. Therapy should be relaxing—not something that causes additional or new pain. Therefore, the initial session of therapeutic traction typically uses less force or weight during distraction (pulling away). The therapist carefully follows cues from the patient relative to the tolerance level, which includes bodily positioning.

Techniques applied in spinal traction are dependent in part on the patient's physical condition, disorder, individual tolerance, and the spinal level(s) to be treated. Application of traction may be manual, positional, or mechanical. Traction may be applied as a continuous force or intermittently. The techniques presented in this section are not all inclusive.

Manual therapeutic traction is a hands-on approach. The patient lies in a relaxed and comfortable position

Spinal traction uses manually or mechanically created forces to stretch and mobilize the spine in an attempt to treat nerve root compression and spine pain.

Nonsurgical Treatment

on the table supine. The therapist carefully positions his hands in such a way to support the patient's head during distraction. The force is gentle, stable, and controlled.

During traction the therapist may reposition the head to one side, flex, or extend the neck using his hands. A change in head position during traction may effect more positive results in reducing the patient's symptoms.

A mechanical traction device used to treat the cervical spine is comprised of a head halter with over-the-door pulley system. Some patients are allowed to use this system at home after the therapist teaches them how to set the system up, wear the halter, apply the weights correctly, and how long to apply the traction. The patient may be able to use the head halter while sitting, reclining, or lying supine.

Manual lumbar traction involves distracting almost half of the body's weight and therefore requires more of the therapist's strength. After the patient is positioned, the therapist may pull at the ankles, once again using controlled force. Another technique involves draping the patient's legs over the therapist's shoulders. The therapist then steadily pulls with his arms positioned across the patient's thighs. An alternative is a pelvic belt with straps used for distraction.

Mechanical traction may incorporate the use of a motorized split-traction table. The patient is placed in a pelvic harness secured to one end of the table. Some motorized units are computerized, enabling the therapist to program the patient's session of therapeutic traction.

When the structural integrity of the spine is compromised (such as in osteoporosis, infection, tumor, or cervical rheumatoid arthritis) traction is not a treatment option. Physical conditions such as pregnancy, cardiovascular disease, hernia, and in some cases temporomandibular joint (TMJ) syndrome exclude patients from spinal traction. In these situations, the forces used in traction (movement) could potentially be dangerous.

82. What can the pain clinic offer me?

Following spinal surgery or if you are not a candidate for spinal surgery, your doctor may refer you to the pain clinic. A pain management assessment begins with your pain history, which includes the location, intensity, and duration of pain as well as factors that alleviate or aggravate pain. A physical and neurological examination is performed. Further, your medical history and test results are reviewed including radiographs (e.g., X-rays, MRI). A multidisciplinary approach means your pain program may include different types of treatment. Treatment is provided by the medical professional who specializes in a specific type of treatment. Medical professionals may include a pain management specialist, physical therapist, rehab specialist, and occupational therapist. Conservative nonsurgical treatment may include a combination of pain-relieving medications, anti-inflammatory drugs, physical therapy, and injections. Alternative therapies include acupuncture, biofeedback, stress reduction, and diet modification.

Nerve blocks are injections of anesthetic, steroid and/or narcotic medications. Nerve blocks are performed to relieve pain and/or to determine if a specific nerve root is the pain source. Anesthetic medications numb the nerves, steroids are potent anti-inflammatory drugs that reduce swelling, and opioids are powerful drugs that fight pain. In some cases, nerve blocks can provide extended periods of pain relief. Some of the different types of nerve blocks are listed next.

- Cervical, thoracic, and lumbosacral medial branch blocks target the medial branch nerves. Medial branch nerves are very small nerves that communicate pain from the spine's facet joints.
- Facet joint blocks are performed to reduce inflammation and pain and to confirm that a particular facet joint is the pain source. The facet joints are small-paired joints on the back of the spine that help to provide spinal stability and guide motion in the back.
- Selective nerve root blocks are performed to reduce inflammation and pain and to determine if a specific nerve root is the pain source.

During the last decade, pain management has evolved into an integral part of patient care that has dramatically affected the medical community. Medical professionals have a better understanding of pain. Attitudes are changing, diagnostic protocols have advanced, technology has improved procedures, and there are more medication options. The horizon continues to brighten for patients who suffer pain.

Richard's comments:

Pain clinic was great for me although ultimately unsuccessful. Again, it was nice having such a dedicated support team to help me through the process, and comforting to know that they were trying everything they could to alleviate my pain and help me avoid surgery.

83. What about IDET, functional discogram, and other nonsurgical treatments for disc disease?

Practically everyone suffers from back pain at some point. Sometimes the pain results from pressure on nerves, sometimes from spinal fractures, and sometimes from problems with the cushioning discs that separate the bones of the spine. Depending on the cause of the pain, treatment can be as simple as rest and exercise or as complex as major surgery. Usually, simpler methods are tried first; if they are not successful in relieving the pain, more aggressive treatments can be used.

A relatively new treatment for back pain resulting from problems within the cushioning discs is intradiscal electrothermal annuloplasty, also called intradiscal electrothermal therapy (IDET). This outpatient procedure applies high heat directly to the inside of the disc. It is a less expensive and less invasive procedure than spinal surgery, but it is not appropriate for everyone who has low back pain.

Discs are cushioning tissues located between each adjoining vertebrae of the spine. The disc has a soft center (nucleus) surrounded by tougher ligament tissue (annulus). As we age, the outer ligament tissue begins to fray and tear from use or injury. This allows nerves and small blood vessels from the soft center to seep into the injury site, triggering pain receptors in the ligament tissue. The result is discogenic back pain.

Discogenic pain differs from a ruptured or herniated disc because the pain originates within the disc and does not come from nerves or other structures. Discogenic pain is confined to the back and does not radiate down the legs.

In addition to interviewing you about the pain, the physician will take your medical history and give you a physical examination. Tests that can help determine the source of the pain include X-rays, magnetic resonance imaging (MRI), computed tomography (CT) scans and discography.

Discography is used to identify the painful disc. In this test, the physician pierces the disc with a thin needle and injects a contrast dye. X-rays show whether the dye enters the disc's outer tissues. Discography is called a provocative test because it will provoke pain in an injured disc.

IDET is usually reserved only for patients who have tried aggressive, nonoperative techniques to relieve their pain without success.

IDET is usually reserved only for patients who have tried aggressive, nonoperative techniques to relieve their pain without success. Because this is a relatively new procedure, you should make sure that the clinician you see is adequately trained in using the equipment. The procedure itself takes about 1 hour to complete. A local anesthetic and intravenous pain relievers are used.

Although IDET is much less invasive than most back surgeries, it will still take several weeks for healing to occur. Pain relief is not immediate; pain may actually increase for a day or 2 after surgery. But gradually the pain from the procedure should diminish.

After the IDET procedure, you will need to rest for a few days and limit the time you spend sitting. You may need to wear a back support for several weeks. You will also need to participate in a physical therapy program. If your job does not involve lifting or manual labor, you may be able to return to work in a week or so; otherwise it may be several months before you can resume your activities. You will not be able to participate in rigorous recreational activity or do any heavy lifting or twisting for at least 6 months after the procedure.

IDET is not recommended if you have severe disc degeneration, nerve compression, spinal instability and/or narrowing of the spinal column (spinal stenosis). IDET is not yet covered by many insurance plans.

The long-term results of this procedure are still unknown. IDET was introduced in 1997 and case series without controls have reported encouraging results. However, these results need to be confirmed in prospective, randomized trials. Additionally, there is debate about how the procedure actually works. Not every patient will benefit from IDET treatment. Some patients continue to experience back pain and may eventually have other surgical procedures.

PART ELEVEN

Surgery on the Spine

What is a discectomy?

What about minimally invasive approaches?

Who should perform my spine surgery?

More ...

84. What is a discectomy?

Intervertebral discs are the soft areas that separate vertebral bodies from each other and provide some shock absorbing capacity to the spine. Also, they allow the spine to be flexible. With age and use the discs become less full of water and can herniated backwards into the spinal cord or spinal roots leading to neurological symptoms.

If a herniated disc causes enough problems and doesn't resolve with conservative management, a discectomy can be performed by your surgeon. A discectomy is the removal of the disc. In the cervical spine, the removed disc is usually replaced with bone. In other parts of the spine the disc can be simply removed without any replacement. The exact surgical plan depends on the disease, patient, and surgeon.

During a lumbar discectomy the patient is placed facedown on the operating table (Figure 36) and an incision is made over the area with the affected disc. A small part of the lamina is removed and using a microscope the lumbar spinal roots and disc are identified. The disc is then removed (Figure 37), freeing up any compression on the lumbar spinal sac and roots. The skin is closed with staples or suture and a dressing is applied.

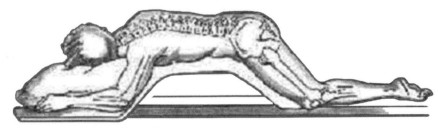

Figure 36   Position of patient in operating room for lumbar microdiscectomy.

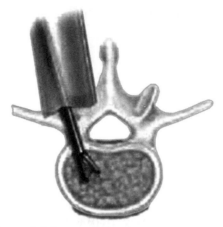

Figure 37   Removal of disc material during surgery.

Richard's comments:

I had my discectomy on my L4 a couple of years ago, and although there were some complications with infection, overall the procedure was a godsend. I found immediate relief for the first couple of days after surgery, but then the pain and numbness came back for a couple of months before they subsided permanently. The doctors said this was due to the swelling of the nerve.

85. What is a decompression?

Decompression is a very general spine term referring to removal of any material causing compression on the spinal nerves or spinal cord. This compressive material is usually a combination of bone, ligaments, joints, and discs. These materials are normally found in the body, but as we age, they may degenerate or herniate, causing compression of neural structures. The most common way to perform a spinal decompression is through a surgical procedure referred to as laminectomy. A laminectomy can be performed with or without a fusion procedure, and it can be performed in the cervical, thoracic, or lumbar spine. A lumbar laminectomy is one of the more common spine procedures.

Lumbar laminectomy is an operation that involves approaching the spine through an incision in the lower back to remove a portion of the bone over and/or around the nerve roots to provide them additional space.

If you have pain caused by pinched nerves, you are a potential candidate for this procedure. While you lie on your stomach (Figure 38), the operation is performed as follows:

- *Incision*—Your surgeon makes an incision in your lower back to access your spine. To have a clear view of your spine, the surgeon then retracts the muscles and ligaments.
- *Bone/disc removal*—Your surgeon removes a portion of the lamina, the bony rim around the spinal canal, if it is contributing to pressure on the dural sac or nerve roots. This part of the procedure is called a laminectomy (Figure 39). The term laminectomy is derived from the Latin words *lamina* (thin plate, sheet, or layer), and *ectomy* (removal). A portion of the bone over the nerve root and/or disc material around the nerve root is removed to give your nerve root additional space.

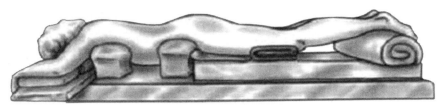

Figure 38   Position of patient in operating room for lumbar fusion.

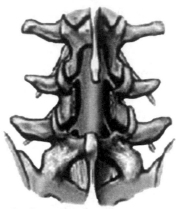

Figure 39   Lumbar laminectomy OK to use.

- *Closure*—The operation is completed when your surgeon closes and dresses the incision. Your surgeon may choose to place a drain into the wound after the surgery to protect the incision.

Your surgeon will have a specific postoperative recovery/ exercise plan to help you return to normal life as soon as possible. The amount of time that you have to stay in the hospital will depend on this treatment plan. By the end of your first day after surgery, you will probably be up and walking in the hospital.

Carrie's comments:

I checked into the hospital on Monday and had my surgery the following morning. The procedure took 13 hours. They made two 6-inch incisions on either side of my spine which I now refer to as my "parentheses." The first part of the procedure was the decompression. This part of my surgery involved a laminectomy or the removal of the part of my L5 that was compressing my spinal cord. This freed up my spinal cord from my slipped L5, and would solve the problem of numbness and paralysis.

86. What is a fusion?

A fusion is the growth of bone over a space or joint. This takes away the ability of the fused bones to move relative to one another. Frequently irregular motion across a degenerated joint or disc space is a major contributor to pain. Also, when a fracture occurs in the spine the safest thing is to create a fusion across that area so no instability occurs.

Recently, significant advancements have been made in the devices and technoligies to achieve fusion in the spine, with smaller and less invasive operations. Further because of biologic agents that are now available the fusions can be created faster and more rigidly. During the fusion process, titanium instrumentation is frequently used to limit movement over the fusing areas in order to allow for the strongest and fastest fusion. This instrumentation which is left inside the wound, doesn't need to be removed and patient can live with it for their lifetimes. On occasion the instrumentation is removed if necessary. See Figure 40.

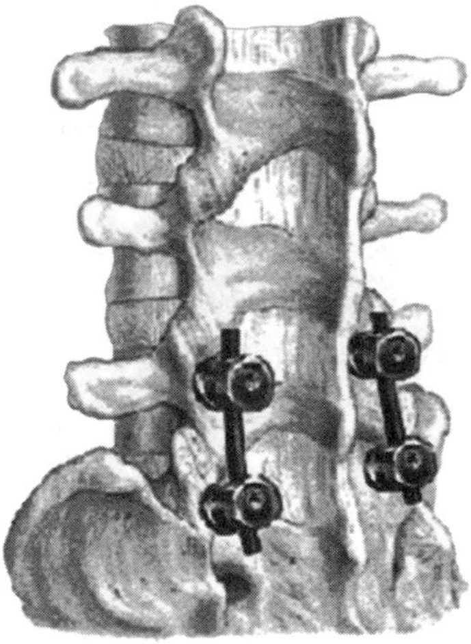

Figure 40   Lumbar spinal fusion with implants.

Carrie's comments:

The second part of my procedure was the spinal fusion. Because of my degenerative spondylolisthesis, they would have to fuse together my L5–S1 to stop the slippage of my L5. To do this, the surgeon took a bone graft from my hip so they could extract bone cells to mix with a cement. This mixture would temporarily hold the fusion in place while at the same time facilitate the growth of new bone cells to form the new bone between my vertebrae. There ended up being more pain from my hip than the actual fusion. The fusion ended up being a complete success and after about a year of recovery, my life was completely back to normal. Indeed, at times I feel like my back is even stronger than most "normal" people have. It's a little weird that I don't ever think about my back any more considering the central role it used to play in my life.

87. What is arthroplasty?

Arthroplasty means artificial joint. Spinal arthroplasty involves replacement of a degenerated spinal disc and placement of an artificial disc. Spinal arthroplasty is investigational in the United States. At the time of this publication, only lumbar arthroplasty has been approved by the Food and Drug Administration (FDA), although several studies are ongoing regarding cervical artificial discs. In more generic terms, spinal arthroplasty encompasses nonfusion techniques surrounding total disc replacement, nucleus (center of the disc) replacement, dynamic stabilization, motion preservation technologies, facet joint replacement, and annulus and nucleus repair and regeneration. Proponents of spinal arthroplasty believe that it will offer significant improvement in pain reduction, reestablishment of a near full range of motion, and restoration of natural disc height, all while keeping the facet joints and surrounding ligament structures and tissues intact.

Arthroplasty

replacing a joint in the body with an artificial joint. In the spine this is most commonly done at the level at which an entire disc is removed and replaced with a prosthetic one, called total disc arthroplasty (TDA).

88. *What about minimally invasive approaches?*

Minimally invasive spine surgery is spine surgery performed through a small incision with the aid of microscopes, endoscopes, or other advanced technology. It has developed out of the desire to treat spine disorders with minimal injury to surrounding tissue. The hope and belief is that this will result in a more rapid recovery. With traditional spine surgery, it may take the body weeks or months to heal. However, with minimally invasive approaches, healing time can substantially be reduced.

It has also been found that minimally invasive approaches, particularly in back surgery, may have other benefits. With traditional back surgery, the surgeon dissects muscles off the spine to access the area of concern. This dissection sometimes results in the loss of innervation (i.e., the supply of nerve stimulation) of the muscles with subsequent wasting away. A permanent weakness of the back muscles may result. This weakness itself may be symptomatic (as a back fatigue-type pain) and/or limit the patient's function, particularly in those who perform physical work.

Clearly, with such significant muscle injury associated with surgical approaches to the spine, the need existed for the development of less invasive surgical techniques. It was envisioned that minimally invasive techniques would offer several advantages, including reduced surgical complications, reduced blood loss, reduced use of postoperative narcotic pain medicines, reduced length of hospital stay, and increased speed of functional return to daily activities. Not all spine disorders can be treated through minimally invasive approaches. However, an increasing number are being treated this way each year.

Carrie's comments:

My surgery was completed about a decade ago, and my understanding is that technology has improved quite a bit since then. I guess surgeries aren't as bad today with lasers and microscopes, and with new endoscopes they can perform operations faster and less invasively. My open surgery was not bad at all. It took half a day and left a couple of big scars, but the initial recovery process was quick, and the final outcome was everything I could have asked for. I would be more concerned with the surgeons being thorough and having full access when working with my spine than be concerned about being quick or minimizing scars.

89. What is spinal instrumentation?

Spinal instrumentation is a generic term referring to implanted devices used during spine surgery. Most of these implants are made of metal (titanium, stainless steel, titanium alloy, etc.) or plastic-like compounds (carbon fiber, polyetheretherketone, etc.). The implants have been tested for safety and used in surgery for decades. Spinal implants are designed for specific purposes and come in many shapes and sizes. Most spinal implants function as a fixation device to allow fusion to occur. They include screws, rods, plates, hooks, cables, and cages. Newer implants, such as artificial discs, are also being developed and tested.

90. What are the risks of surgery?

The risks of surgery depend entirely on the type of surgery you are going to have. With any surgery, no mater how small there are inherent risks or bleeding, infection, and on a very rare occasion death. The degree to which these risks are for your particular surgery is something you should discuss at length with your surgeon. Below are some risks that should be discussed.

- *Complication of anesthesia*
- *Risk of bleeding*
- *Risk of infection*
- *Risk of death*
- *Risk of blood clots in your legs after surgery*
- *Risk of spinal cord or root injury*
- *Risk of tear in the dura and post-surgery spinal fluid leak*
- *Chance of persistent pain after surgery*
- *Chance of problems with failure in the instrumentation used*
- *Chance for need of reoperation*

Richard's comments:

Risk of infection is real! After my surgery, the surgeons told me everything went fine, but then I got an infection and was in the hospital for another 5 days. I got a bad infection in my back and had to get a PICC [peripherally inserted central catheter] line into my arm so I could inject IV fluids every 8 hours at home. There were more complications with my infection and the PICC line, and I had to go to the ER twice. It stayed in for 5 weeks.

91. Who should perform my spine surgery?

There is much debate about what type of physician should perform spine surgery. Spine surgery in the United States is performed by neurosurgeons and orthopedic surgeons. A neurosurgeon is a physician who completed a 7-year training program following medical school in the surgical management of disorders of the brain, spine, and peripheral nerves. He or she may have also completed a 1-year fellowship specifically dealing with disorders of the spine. An orthopedic surgeon is a physician who completed a 5-year training program following medical school in the surgical and nonsurgical management of disorders of the bones, joints, and musculoskeletal system. Orthopedic spine surgeons have generally completed a 1-year fellowship specifically dealing with disorders of the spine.

Regardless of specialty, the most important thing is that your surgeon is board certified or board eligible and routinely performs the procedure he or she is recommending for you. In addition, he or she should be trained to treat any potential complication that may be encountered. Be sure to ask your doctor if he or she is board certified or board eligible, and how often he or she performs your specific type of spine surgery. If you have any doubt, get a second opinion.

Carrie's comments:

I had my surgery performed by a neurosurgical spine specialist. As a neurosurgeon and spine specialist, he was highly regarded by my referring physician, and a bit of online research confirmed [his qualifications]. Because he was a neurosurgeon, I felt he paid particular attention to my spinal cord, and my neurological outcomes maybe more than an orthopedic surgeon would have. He was very knowledgeable and confident, but at the same time comforting, but was also able to ease my anxiety and gain my trust by keeping me completely in the know about everything else.

92. What about the future of spine surgery?

The future of spine surgery is promising. As our population ages, more and more people will likely be in need of treatment for a spine disorder. Efforts are under way to improve minimally invasive techniques, designed to lessen the risks and hardships of surgery and speed the recovery process. Arthroplasty, or artificial disc technology, is likely to become a larger component of spine surgery, and is used more frequently to treat certain spinal ailments. In addition, certain biologic agents that may reverse the damage to nerves, cartilage, discs, and bones that occur as we age are being investigated, thus reducing the need for surgery altogether.

Richard's comments:

At the time of my surgery, I was offered the option of trying a minimally invasive correction, but felt that it was still best to take an open approach since I wasn't too concerned about scarring. I have heard that since then the frontier of spine surgery has largely shifted in this direction and minimally invasive and endoscopic techniques are honed and perfected. Also, things like radiosurgery and stem cell therapeutics are on the horizon and constantly in the news. They all seem like exciting developments to me.

PART TWELVE

Spine Rehabilitation

What are my limitations?

How long do I have to wear my collar or brace?

What about pain management?

More ...

93. How long is rehabilitation after surgery?

The rehabilitation after surgery is directly related to the reason you are having surgery, how extensive the surgery is, and if you have any complications from surgery. Some patients go home the same day after spine surgery and others will require days to weeks. If complications arise the stay could be longer depending on the complication. The great majority of patients don't have complications and do very well.

After the operation you will recover initially in the recovery room where your pain will be controlled and the anesthetic will be allowed to wear off. Subsequently, you will be taken to your hospital room and allowed to eat and drink as you can tolerate. Your activity level depends on your disease and surgery, but most people will be encouraged to walk the next day in order to minimize complications and this may or may not be with a brace (decided by your surgeon). Also, on the first day after surgery your incision may be evaluated by removing the dressing. Some types of spine surgery require the placement of drains in the wound that drain outside and these may be evaluated and/or removed as well.

Both in the hospital and as an outpatient you may work closely with a physical therapist to maximize your quick and safe return to full activity. While at home you will have specific instructions on care for your incision and reasons that you should call your physician.

For the first several weeks strenuous activity is restricted and most spine surgery patients are asked no to lift or carry objects heavier than 5 pounds. With gradual increase of activity and physical therapy most patients return to work within weeks. As stated earlier the recovery is dependent on the spine disease and spine surgery, but as an example patients after a lumbar discectomy for herniated disc go home the day after surgery and usually return to work the second week after discharge from the hospital.

Carrie's comments:

For my spinal decompression and fusion, the entire recovery process took about a year. It was probably several more after that before my back was completely pain free and at 100% strength. They had me on my feet using a walker a couple of days after the surgery, and I was discharged by the end of the week. I spent most of the next 3 months on my back with a brace on to allow for new bone growth to occur and the fusion to set. For half a year after that I wore a corset-like brace, my back was weak, and I still felt pain for at least a year after my surgery. But with time I soon realized positive results. Now years after my procedure, I seldom have back pain except when I work out especially hard. Though it may take awhile to realize the results are truly positive, and I'm glad to say that the back pain era of my life is definitely behind me.

94. When can I go back to work?

When you go back to work depends, in large part, on what you do at work and what type of procedure you have done. For example, if you have an office job and undergo a lumbar discectomy, you may be back at work in as short as 1–2 weeks. However, if your work requires heavy lifting (such as construction work), and you have a more involved procedure such as lumbar fusion for a spine fracture, you may be out of work for several months. In addition, the rate at which individuals heal following surgery is not identical. In general, older patients require a longer time to heal, as do those with other medical problems (e.g., diabetes).

Carrie's comments:

After the initial 3 months in bed, I was able to venture back out into the world with a corset brace without any major problems, although any physically demanding activities were out of the question.

95. What are my limitations?

Limitations following surgery are also dependent upon the procedure you have done. In general, however, limitations come in three categories:

1. Wound limitations
2. Spine limitations
3. General limitations

Wound limitations are imposed until the wound has fully healed. This includes proper wound care. Limitations would include swimming, soaking in a bath, applying lotions on or near the wound, getting a tattoo near the wound, etc. All these may lead to infection. Once the wound has entirely healed (between 2 and 6 weeks) these limitations are generally lifted.

Spine limitations may include avoidance of lifting objects more than 10 pounds, twisting motions (such as a golf swing or tennis stroke), avoiding excessive bending, etc. These limitations are imposed until your spine has healed. The time it takes for healing to occur depends upon the procedure you have, but takes generally anywhere from 6 weeks to 3 months. Spinal rehabilitation is generally started at 6 weeks after surgery, but limitations may be in place for several months after surgery.

General limitations refer to activities that should be modified as a result of suffering from a spine disorder or avoidance of a future spinal disorder. This is a very broad category but includes ergonomic modifications at home and work. For example, a jackhammer operator may need to find different work following some types of back surgery even if the wound is completely healed. Another example would be a patient who has a cervical laminectomy; he or she would be advised not to ride roller coasters. These limitations are broad and depend upon the nature of your disease and the treatment you had done.

Carrie's comments:

Now that I have fully recovered, my back is at 100% strength. Indeed, at times because I work out and stay fit, my back feels stronger than most "normal" people's backs probably do. I have returned to all the activities that I love including backpacking, cross-country skiing, and running. I know there are a lot of scary stories about spine surgery out there, but there are far more success stories like mine. If the procedure wasn't successful, they wouldn't continue performing it year after year. If I had a choice to do the fusion again or not, I would not hesitate to go for it.

96. What about adjacent level disease?

Patients who have disease at one level in the spine are at higher risk of having problems at other levels. Most commonly, the next adjacent level is at higher risk. The exact reason for this is not entirely known, but the thought is that a degenerated level does not work properly and, as result, places greater strain on the next level of the spine. Many believe this adjacent level phenomenon is accentuated following certain types of fusion surgery since normal motion is stopped and the next level needs to accommodate excessive motion. This has been shown to be the case in laboratory studies but has not definitely been shown to be the case clinically. Regardless, the risk of adjacent level disease is one argument in favor of arthroplasty (artificial disk placement) instead of fusion to treat certain types of spine problems. Time will tell if arthroplasty truly reduces the incidence of adjacent level disease.

97. How long do I have to wear my collar or brace?

The length of time you have to wear your collar or brace is determined by the nature of the injury you suffered, the surgery (if any) you had to correct it, and the rate at which your body heals. For most types of whiplash without any fracture, a collar is worn for 2 to 6 weeks. Following routine cervical surgery, a collar is rarely worn for more than 6 weeks. In the case of a fracture (particularly an odontoid fracture) that was not treated with surgery, a collar may need to be worn for as long as 3 months. Your doctor will order periodic X-rays to assess bone healing. This will play a major factor in determining how long a collar or brace needs to be worn.

Carrie's comments:

I wore my brace for a total of 9 months. I spent 3 months with a hyperextension brace on my back to allow for new bone growth to ensure that the fusion stabilized. Then I had to wear a different rigid lumbar brace for another 6 months. The first 3 months were particularly hard because I missed out on a lot of things being basically confined to the bed. For an entire year after that I was back out again, but the brace made it hard to do what I usually enjoy doing since I was a pretty active person before my surgery. It was a difficult process, but ultimately worth it.

98. What is a bone stimulator?

A bone stimulator is a device worn outside the skin designed to stimulate bone growth after surgery or trauma. The device works by transmitting a low-voltage electrical current. The devices do not require surgical implantation or extraction. Typically, the device is worn after spine fusion either as small, thin skin pads/electrodes that are placed directly over the fusion site or as coils placed into a brace.

Unlike an internal (implanted) bone growth stimulator, an external bone growth stimulator may also be prescribed for the patient to use several weeks or months after the fusion surgery if the bone is not fusing as desired.

Depending on the device and the patient's situation, an external bone growth stimulator will be prescribed to be worn for a specific number of hours each day (typically within the range of 2–9 hours per day). Sometimes the patient may be allowed to break it up into several 1- or 2-hour sessions each day, or to vary the times that the device is worn each day, to better suit the patient's schedule. Typically, the external bone growth stimulator will be worn for a period of 3–9 months following the surgery.

An external electrical stimulator is usually lightweight and powered by a battery, so it is very portable. Patients may move about and complete their daily activities as they normally would with the device. However, the surgeon may restrict the patient's activities due to the fusion surgery, and there are some activities for which the patient should remove the device (e.g., swimming, bathing).

As with the internal stimulators, the external device is not painful and the patient cannot feel any electrical shocks or vibrations while wearing it.

While external electrical stimulation devices are considered very safe, it is important to note that the electromagnetic effects of this type of treatment are unknown for pregnant women and for some types of pacemakers and defibrillators.

A theoretical disadvantage of an external stimulator versus the internal stimulator is that there may be less patient compliance with wearing the external stimulator the required number of hours. Obviously, if the patient does not wear the device, the benefits from the treatment will not be realized.

A potential advantage of external stimulators versus internal stimulators is that the external device is usually a less expensive treatment option and does not require the potential second surgery to remove the battery pack.

Another major advantage is that an external bone stimulator can be added after the fusion has been done if there is concern that the bone graft is not healing and a nonunion is developing.

99. What if I'm a smoker?

Smoking is known to reduce the rate of bone fusion following surgery or trauma. The exact mechanism of this is not known, but many suspect decreased blood supply to bones as the culprit. Regardless, if you are a

Smoking is known to reduce the rate of bone fusion following surgery or trauma.

smoker and in need of spine surgery, your physician may insist that you quit smoking for a period of time before and after surgery in order to optimize the chance that surgery will be successful. Other alternatives include using autograft (bone from another part of the same person's body) for spine surgery instead of allograft (bone from a cadaver) or titanium. Also, BMP (bone morphogenic protein) has been shown to increase rates for fusion. Regardless, smoking is associated with higher risk of nonunion (bones that do not heal) and wound healing issues. Speak with your surgeon about the additional risks of surgery for smokers.

100. What about pain management?

Pain management is often a major component of treating a spinal disorder. For some, meeting with a pain management specialist begins well before surgery is ever considered. For others, aggressive pain management is the final option after having extinguished every other option, including surgery.

Pain management physicians are anesthesiologists who specialize in administration of pain medications, injections for complex pain, and interventional procedures to treat pain (e.g., narcotic intrathecal pump). They may also help isolate precisely the location from where pain is coming.

Richard's comments:

Pain management is a great idea if you are recovering from surgery or are in some other way in continuous pain. But the most debilitating aspect of my back pain was that it was unpredictable and intermittent. Even though I was able to manage the pain, it was a sporadic process that really disrupted my life.

Glossary

Arthritis: Normal aging and wear and tear on bones and joints causes inflammation and pain referred to as arthritis. This can occur at any joint in the body and is common in the joints of the neck and low back.

Arthrodesis: Fusion of bones. In the spine, one or more vertebrae are often fused together in order to stop pain and compression of nerves and the spinal cord.

Arthroplasty: Replacing a joint in the body with an artificial joint. In the spine this is most commonly done at the level at which an entire disc is removed and replaced with a prosthetic one, called total disc arthroplasty (TDA).

Benign: A tumor that is not cancerous or malignant. Benign lesions can still grow and cause damage to surrounding structures.

Cancer: A condition in which there is an uncontrolled growth of cells that spread throughout the body.

CAT scan; CT scan: Abbreviations for computerized axial tomography (CAT) or computed tomography (CT) scan. A noninvasive diagnostic test that relies on X-rays and computerized reconstruction to image parts of the body. This technique is very quick and very good for looking at bone and dense instructions of the body.

Cervical: The neck region. Specifically, there are seven cervical vertebrae in the human spine. They are numbered C1, C2, etc. The nerves that exit the spine in this region are responsible for movement and sensation in the arms and hands.

Congenital: A disease that came prior to birth. This is opposed to degenerative, which occurs as one ages.

Decompression: The removal of bone, disc, cartilage, ligament, or a tumor that is compressing on the spinal cord or nerve routes. Decompression surgery is often performed in conjunction with fusion if the amount of decompression is likely to cause spinal instability.

Degenerative: The changes that occur with normal aging. Degenerative diseases generally progress slowly.

Disc: The soft, gelatinous material that acts as a cushion between vertebrae in the spine. As we age, the disc degenerates or herniates and is often the source of back or neck pain.

Discogram: A test in which dye is injected in the disc to determine if there is a disc disruption or to determine if a particular disc is the source of back or neck pain.

Epidural: The space above and around the dura, which is the sac that contains the spinal cord and nerves. It is a place where medication can be delivered to treat back or neck pain.

Facet: The medical term for the spinal joint. Each vertebra has two facets, one on each site. The facets are often the source of pain for people with low back pain.

Herniation: Condition that occurs when a material (usually a disc) squeezes out of its intended place. The herniated disc fragment often compresses an adjacent nerve or the spinal cord, causing pain or neurologic injury.

Instrumentation: The placement of foreign material used to fuse or aid in the structure of the spine. Most instrumentation involves titanium rods and screws that are implanted in

the spine and hold it in proper position while healing or arthrodesis occurs.

Lumbar: The low back region. Specifically, there are five lumbar vertebrae in the human spine. They are numbered L1, L2, etc. The nerves that exit the spine in this region are responsible for movement and sensation in the legs and feet.

Malignant: A tumor that is cancerous or has the potential to spread to another part of the body. Tumors vary with respect to how malignant or aggressive they are.

Metastasis: The spread of cancer cells from their original site to other locations.

MRI: Abbreviation for magnetic resonance imaging. A noninvasive diagnostic test that uses high-powered magnets to image parts of the body. This technique is very good at looking at soft tissues of the body, such as the spinal cord, discs, ligaments, and muscles.

Myelogram: A test in which dye is injected into the spinal sac around the spinal cord and various X-rays are taken. The test is often used to evaluate for spinal compression in patients who cannot undergo MRI.

Occipital: A term used to refer to the back and bottom part of the skull. This is the part of the skull that is in contact with the top of the spine.

Osteopenia: A decrease in bone mineral density that occurs in some people as they age. It can be a precursor to osteoporosis, though not everyone with osteopenia develops osteoporosis.

Osteoporosis: A bone condition in which bone mineral density is reduced substantially and bone collagen is disrupted. Bones become weaker and people with the condition are at higher risk of developing a fracture.

Radiation therapy: Treatment of disease by means of X-rays or of radioactive substances.

Scoliosis: A spinal disorder in which the spine develops abnormal lateral and rotational curvature. In severe cases, walking, complex movements, and even breathing can be compromised.

Spina bifida: A developmental spinal birth defect in which the primitive spinal column does not properly close while the embryo is in utero. Children with this defect are born with varying degrees of closure and varying degrees of spinal cord damage from extremely mild to complete paralysis.

Spinal cord: The nervous system tissue that relays information to and from the limbs and the brain. It is located within the center of and protected by the vertebrae.

Spondylectomy: The complete removal of a spinal vertebra through a surgical procedure. It is commonly performed for removal of a tumor. Following spondylectomy, the spine is usually stabilized with hardware.

Spondylosis: Arthritis of the spine. It is associated with normal and abnormal motion of vertebrae over time.

Spondylolisthesis: A condition in which one vertebra slides out of position with respect to an adjacent vertebra. This most commonly occurs in the lumbar spine and is gradual and progressive in nature.

Stenosis: Narrowing of the spinal canal. It can occur gradually over time or acutely when a disc herniates or a vertebra fractures. If the narrowing is severe, then critical structures within the canal, such as nerves and the spinal cord, can be compressed, causing neurologic injury.

Thoracic: The mid-back region. Specifically, there are twelve thoracic vertebrae in the human spine, each associated with a pair of ribs. They are numbered T1, T2, etc.

Urodynamics: A series of tests used to evaluate the neurological function of the urinary system. Severe injury to the low back may cause urinary problems and urodynamics may help assess the degree of damage.

Vertebra: One segment of the spine. The spine is comprised of seven cervical vertebrae, twelve thoracic vertebrae, and five lumbar vertebrae.

Index

Index

Index

Index

T

T-score, 49
tethered spinal cord syndrome, 97, 99
thoracic disc herniation, symptoms
    of, 23
thoracic spine
    braces for, 63, 125–127
    defined. *See* stability of spine
    injury to, 75. *See also* spinal cord
        injury
    spinal cord level, 12
thoracic vertebrae, 4
tobacco use, 159–160
traction, 129–131
transverse process fractures, 59
trauma to spine. *See* spine trauma
traumatic spondylolisthesis, 42
treatment
    basilar invagination, 45
    burst fracture, 54
    cervical spondylosis, 33–34
    compression fracture (wedge
        fracture), 51
    healing time for spinal fractures,
        64–65
    herniated discs, 25–28
    nonsurgical. *See* conservative
        treatment
    odontoid fracture, 55
    rehabilitation, 153–160
    scoliosis, 90–91, 92–93
    spinal stenosis, 38–39
    spine tumors, 84–86
    spondylolisthesis, 42–43
    surgical. *See* surgery (as treatment)
tumors, 81–86
    diagnosing, 84
    metastatic disease, 83–84
    treatment, 84–86

U

urinary tract problems, patients with
    SCI, 76
urodynamics, 100–101

V

vascular claudication, 37–38
ventilator-dependent quadriplegia,
    74
ventral roots (spinal nerves), 8
vertebra, first (atlas), 44
vertebrae, 4
    defined, 5
    dislocation of, 57–59, 62
    removal of (spondylectomy),
        85–86
vertebral arch, 4, 5–6
vertebral bodies, 4–5
    degeneration of intervertebral
        discs, 15
vertebral body
    dislocation of, 57–59, 62
    slippage forward. *See*
        spondylolisthesis
vertebral fractures
    burst fracture, 52–54
    compression fracture (wedge
        fracture), 50–52
    hangman's fracture, 56–57
    Jefferson's fracture, 57
    odontoid fracture, 54–56
vertebral levels, 12

W

weakness from spine fracture,
    60
wedge fracture. *See* compression
    fracture
weight bearing. *See* stability of spine
weight control, patients with SCI,
    76
work after surgery, 154–155
wound limitations following surgery,
    155
wounds in patients with SCI, 74, 75,
    76

X

X-rays, 106–108